D1125361

PRINCIPLES AND
PRACTICE OF
INFECTIOUS DISEASES

Antimicrobial
Therapy
1992

PRINCIPLES AND PRACTICE OF INFECTIOUS DISEASES

Antimicrobial Therapy 1992

Gerald L. Mandell, M.D.
R. Gordon Douglas, Jr., M.D.
John E. Bennett, M.D.

Churchill Livingstone
New York, Edinburgh, London, Melbourne, Tokyo

Library of Congress Cataloging-in-Publication Data

Mandell, Gerald L.
    Principles and practice of infectious diseases, antimicrobial
therapy / Gerald L. Mandell, R. Gordon Douglas, Jr.,
John E. Bennett.
      p.   cm.
    Companion v. to: Principles and practice of infectious diseases /
edited by Gerald L. Mandell, R. Gordon Douglas, Jr., John E.
Bennett. 3rd ed. 1990.
    ISBN 0-443-08818-7
    1. Anti-infective agents—Handbooks, manuals, etc. I. Douglas,
R. Gordon (Robert Gordon), date.   II. Bennett, John E. (John
Eugene), date.   III. Principles and practice of infectious
diseases. IV. Title.
    [DNLM: 1. Communicable Diseases—therapy—handbooks. WC 39 M271p]
RM267.M26 1992
616.9'046—dc20
DNLM/DLC
for Library of Congress   91-36236
                                                             CIP

Distributed in the United Kingdom by Churchill Livingstone, Robert Stevenson
House, 1–3 Baxter's Place, Leith Walk, Edinburgh EH1 3AF, and by associated com-
panies, branches, and representatives throughout the world.

Every effort has been made to provide accurate indications, and dosage schedules for
drugs. The reader is urged to review the package information data of the manufacturers
of the medications mentioned.

The Publishers have made every effort to trace the copyright holders for borrowed
material. If they have inadvertently overlooked any, they will be pleased to make the
necessary arrangements at the first opportunity.

Acquisitions Editor: *Robert A. Hurley*
Production Designer: *Alice Cheung*
Production Supervisor: *Christina Hippeli*

Printed in the United States of America

First published in 1992   7 6 5 4 3

Introduction

Many physicians have requested a pocket-sized companion book to our comprehensive infectious disease textbook, *Principles and Practice of Infectious Diseases*. To fulfill that request, we wrote this handbook to provide rapid, concise, and up-to-date guidance for therapy of known or presumed infectious diseases. Although the handbook is not meant to be a comprehensive reference, it should be used as an aid in making therapeutic decisions. Consult *Principles and Practice of Infectious Diseases* for more in-depth coverage.

The *first section* is an overview of antimicrobial agents by class that allows discussion of antimicrobial agent properties to be presented most efficiently. The *second section* is an extensive table of empiric therapy for infectious syndromes that closely follows the organization of Part Two (Major Clinical Syndromes) in *Principles and Practice of Infectious Diseases*. This section uses an organ system approach. Organisms likely to cause these syndromes are listed and effective antimicrobial programs are presented. *Section three* considers therapy for infections caused by identified organisms. Parasitic diseases often seen in the United States and industrialized countries are included. *Section four* outlines therapy for sexually transmitted diseases. Therapy of HIV associated infections is discussed in *section five*. *Section six* is a consideration of prophylactic uses of antimicrobial agents. *Section seven* lists the indicated and contraindicated agents to pregnancy. *Section eight* consists of a series of tables of pertinent pharmacologic features of antimicrobial agents and *section nine* lists generic and trade names of antimicrobial drugs. We will revise this handbook yearly and welcome your comments and suggestions.

Gerald L. Mandell, M.D.
R. Gordon Douglas, Jr., M.D.
John E. Bennett, M.D.

Rapid Guide

1. For information concerning treatment of an infectious syndrome consult Section 2—organized by organ system.

2. For properties and doses of antimicrobial agents consult Section 8—organized alphabetically by generic name (see Section 9 for generic/trade and trade/generic lists).

3. For agents effective for specific pathogens consult Section 3—organized alphabetically by microbe.

Table of Contents

Section 1

SUMMARY OF ANTIMICROBIAL AGENTS BY CLASS

ANTIBACTERIAL AGENTS

Penicillins

Classification of Penicillins

Natural Penicillins	Penicillin G Aqueous Procaine Benzathine Penicillin V Phenethicillin
Penicillinase-resistant penicillins (anti-staphylococcal penicillins)	Methicillin Nafcillin Isoxazolyl penicillins Cloxacillin Dicloxacillin Flucloxacillin Oxacillin
Aminopenicillins	Ampicillin Amoxicillin Bacampicillin Cyclacillin Hetacillin
Anti-Pseudomonas penicillins	Azlocillin Carbenicillin Carbenicillin indanyl sodium Ticarcillin Mezlocillin Piperacillin

Antimicrobial Activities

Penicillin G is active against most aerobic gram-positive organisms and is more active than the semisynthetic penicillins versus gram-positive cocci. Penicillin V generally can be used as a well-absorbed oral substitute for penicillin G. Ampicillin and amoxicillin have some activity versus several gram-negative rods, and the gram-negative spectrum is increased with carbenicillin and ticarcillin and more so with azlocillin, mezlocillin, and piperacillin. Most anaerobes are susceptible to penicillins, with the notable exception of *Bacteroides fragilis*, which is sensitive only to the anti-*Pseudomonas* penicillins.

Resistance - Mechanism

Enzymatic hydrolysis by β-lactamases
    Gram-positive bacteria - plasmid mediated
    Gram-negative bacteria - chromosome or plasmid mediated
Failure to reach receptor site
    Gram-negative bacteria - alteration in membrane properties

Pharmacokinetics

Many penicillins are acid labile and not well-absorbed after oral administration. Peak blood levels occur early—1 to 2 hours after oral ingestion and immediately with intravenous administration. They are variably protein bound (17 to 97%). Penicillins are rapidly excreted by the kidney, resulting in a short half-life. The primary mechanism is excretion by renal tubular cells, which accounts for up to 4 g/hr. Renal excretion can be blocked by probenecid, and is less in newborns. In the presence of anuria, the dosage of most penicillins must be modified. Penicillins penetrate many body spaces and fluids in sufficient quantities to inhibit micro-organisms, but penetration of the eye, brain, cerebrospinal fluid (CSF), and prostate is very low in the absence of inflammation.

Adverse Effects

Hypersensitivity reactions occur in 0.7 to 4% of patients treated with any one of the penicillins. There is no difference among them with regard to potential for causing such effects. Anaphylactic reactions, which are the most serious

Antimicrobial Activity of Penicillins

	Penicillin G	Ampicillin Amoxicillin	Oxacillin Nafcillin	Carbenicillin Ticarcillin	Azlocillin Mezlocillin Piperacillin
Streptococcus pyogenes	++++	++++	++++	++	++++
Streptococcus pneumoniae	++++	++++	++++	++	++++
Enterococcus faecalis	+	++	—	—	++
Staphylococcus aureus					
Penase-negative	++++	++++	++++	++	++
Penase-positive	—	—	++++	—	—
Neisseria gonorrhoeae Pen-susceptible	++++	++++	—	++	++++
Neisseria meningitidis	++++	++++	—	++	++++
Haemophilus influenzae β-lactamase negative strains	—	++	—	++	++++
Escherichia coli	—	+	—	++	++
Proteus mirabilis	—	++	—	++	+++
Proteus, other	—	—	—	+	+
Klebsiella spp.	—	—	—	—	+
Enterobacter spp.	—	—	—	+	+
Serratia	—	—	—	—	—
Pseudomonas aeruginosa	—	—	—	+	+
Acinetobacter	—	—	—	+	++

+ to ++++ indicates degree of activity; — indicates inactivity.

because they may cause sudden death, occur in 0.004 to 0.015% of persons treated with a penicillin, and death due to such reactions is about once in every 50,000 to 100,000 treatment courses.

Hypersensitivity reactions are due to antibodies directed against the major and minor determinants. The penicilloyl moiety, formed when the β-lactam ring is opened, is the major determinant. The intact molecule itself, penicilloate, and other breakdown products constitute the minor determinants. Immediate allergic reactions are mediated by IgE antibodies to the minor determinant, whereas accelerated and late urticarial reaction results from major determinant-specific antibodies. Maculopapular reactions may be due to immune complexes involving IgM antibodies.

Adverse effects may include the following:

Hypersensitivity reactions
    Most common
        Maculopapular rash
        Urticarial rash
        Fever
        Bronchospasm
    Less common
        Vasculitis
        Coombs reaction
        Neutropenia
        Interstitial nephritis
        Serum sickness
        Exfoliative dermatitis
        Stevens-Johnson syndrome
        Toxic epidermal necrolysis
        Angioedema
        Anaphylaxis
Toxic effects
    Most common
        Gastrointestinal symptoms with oral forms
    Less common
        Bone marrow depression, granulocytopenia
        Hepatitis
        Impairment in platelet aggregation (penicillin G, carbenicillin, ticarcillin)

Focal myoclonus
Seizures
Local reactions to intermuscular injection

Management of the Potentially Allergic Patient

If the patient has a history of allergy to penicillin:
Use another antibiotic, preferably not a β-lactam (aztreonam may be the exception).

If above is not possible, skin test (for procedure and interpretation, see *Principles and Practice of Infectious Diseases*, page 264).

If patient is allergic and penicillin *must* be given, desensitize the patient using gradually increasing doses of penicillin. This is rarely necessary and may be dangerous. (See *Principles and Practice of Infectious Diseases* for details.)

Cephalosporins and Cephamycins

Mechanism of Action and Resistance

Cephalosporins inhibit bacterial cell wall synthesis in a fashion similar to penicillins. The major mechanism of resistance is due to the action of β-lactamases which hydrolyze the β-lactam ring required for antimicrobial activity. There is marked variation in susceptibility among cephalosporins to β-lactamases, with cephalothin being most resistant to hydrolysis by β-lactamases produced by *S. aureus* and cefoxitin, cefuroxime, and third generation cephalosporins most resistant to those produced by gram-negative rods.

Adverse Effects

Hypersensitivity reactions
    Most common
        Maculopapular rash
        Urticarial rash
        Fever
    Less common
        Eosinophilia
        Positive Coombs reaction

Pharmacokinetic Properties of Cephalosporins

Oral Preparations	IV Only	IM or IV	CSF Penetration
Cephalexin	Cephalothin	Cefazolin	Cefuroxime
Cephradine	Cephapirin	Cefamandole	Cefotaxime
Cefaclor		Cefoxitin	Ceftriaxone
Cefadroxil		Cefuroxime	Ceftizoxime
Cefuroxime axetil		Cefonicid[a]	Ceftazidime
Cefixime[a]		Cefotetan[a]	
		Ceforanide[a]	
		Cefotaxime	
		Ceftizoxime	
		Ceftriaxone[b]	
		Cefoperazone[c]	
		Ceftazidime	
		Cefmetazole	
		Moxalactam	

[a]Extended half-life.
[b]Very extended half-life.
[c]Decrease dose in hepatic failure.

Adverse Effects (continued from page 6)

Bronchospasm
Anaphylaxis
Toxic effects
Nephrotoxicity - rare
Diarrhea
Intolerance to alcohol (cefamandole, cefotetan, moxalactam, cefoperazone, cefmetazole)
Bleeding (moxalactam)
Hypoprothrombinemia
Thrombocytopenia
Platelet dysfunction

Classification of Cephalosporins

Generation	Members	Activity
First	Cephalothin Cefazolin Cephapirin Cephalexin Cephradine Cefadroxil	Most gram-positive cocci, (except enterococci, MRSA, *S. epidermidis*) *E. coli, Klebsiella pneumoniae, Pr. mirabilis*
Second	Cefamandole Cefaclor Cefuroxime Cefonicid Ceforanide	Less active against gram-positive cocci than first generation More active against *some* gram-negative organisms, especially *H. influenzae, Enterobacter* species, indole-positive *Proteus* species
	Cefoxitin Cefotetan Cefmetazole	Less active against gram-positive cocci than first generation More active against *some* gram-negative organisms Significant activity against anaerobes including *B. fragilis*
Third	Cefotaxime Ceftizoxime Ceftriaxone	Expanded activity against gram-negative rods Poor activity against *B. fragilis* Slightly less active against gram-positive cocci than first generation
	Cefoperazone Ceftazidime	Above properties of third generation cephalosporins but even less active against gram-positive cocci Activity against *Pseudomonas aeruginosa*
	Cefixime	Above properties of third generation cephalosporins but even less active against gram-positive cocci Not active against *Pseudomonas aeruginosa*

Other β-Lactam Antibiotics

Carbapenems

Imipenem is a carbapenem, a class of compounds closely related to, but chemically distinct from, the penicillins, cephalosporins, and cephamycins. It has excellent activity against most gram-positive and gram-negative aerobic and anaerobic pathogens, the notable exceptions being *Pseudomonas cepacia*, *Xanthomonas maltophilia*, and methicillin-resistant *Staphylococcus aureus*. It is given intravenously in equal parts with cilastatin, an inhibitor of dehydropeptidase, a renal enzyme that hydrolyzes imipenem.

Adverse Effects of Imipenem

Allergic reactions
ALT, AST elevations
Leukopenia
Seizures in patients with underlying central nervous system (CNS) disease and/or impaired renal function

Monobactams

Aztreonam

Aztreonam is active against aerobic gram-negative rods and is similar to aminoglycosides in that respect. It can be used in patients allergic to other β-lactam antibiotics because of its different antigenic properties.

β-Lactamase Inhibitors

Clavulanate and sulbactam are β-lactamase inhibitors. If combined with a penicillin the spectrum of antimicrobial activity of the penicillin is extended.

When combined with amoxicillin, clavulanate does not alter the pharmacokinetics of amoxicillin or contribute to increased side-effects. However, it enhances the antimicrobial spectrum to include not only β-lactamase producing *Haemophilus influenzae* and *Moraxella catarrhalis*, but also staphylococci, *Neisseria gonorrhoeae, E. coli, K. pneumoniae, Proteus* sp., and *B. fragilis.*

Combining clavulanate with ticarcillin produces an enhanced spectrum against certain gram-positive and gram-negative organisms.

Sulbactam is chemically related to clavulanate. When added to ampicillin or cefoperazone, it has enhanced the antibacterial spectrum of the parent compounds.

Aminoglycosides and Spectinomycin: Aminocyclitols

Antimicrobial Activity

Aminoglycosides are active primarily against aerobic and facultative gram-negative bacilli and *S. aureus*. In spite of differences in in vitro sensitivity among the aminoglycosides, there is no evidence to indicate that one is superior to the others in a clinical situation against a susceptible organism. Streptomycin is effective against *M. tuberculosis, Francisella tularensis, Yersinia pestis,* and *Brucella* sp. Kanamycin is limited in its spectrum. Gentamicin, tobramycin, and netilmicin are active against a broad range of gram-negative organisms, while amikacin has an even broader range of activity.

Resistance

Ribosomal resistance is uncommmon and pertains to streptomycin
Ineffective transport
Enzymatic degradation of aminoglycoside - most common
    Conjugation with acetyl group
    Conjugation with adenyl group
    Conjugation with phosphoryl group
Enzymes are plasmid-mediated and multiple enzymes exist
Amikacin is the most resistant to enzymatic degradation, hence its broad
    spectrum of activity

Pharmacokinetic Properties

After intravenous or intramuscular administration, peak levels are reached in 30 minutes to 1 hour. The half-life is 1.5 to 3.5 hours, with excretion entirely by the kidneys. Blood levels fall so that repeat doses must be given at 8- to 12-hour intervals.

Because of the frequency of dose-related toxicity and the narrow range between therapeutic and toxic levels, blood levels should be monitored while aminoglycosides are being administered. Age of patient, presence of disease states, and other factors affect dosing. In infants, larger than usual adult doses on a mg/kg basis are used due to an increased volume of distribution. In the elderly, longer half-lives necessitate longer dosing intervals or lower doses. Dosage modification is required for renal impairment. Obesity, malnutrition, fever, and burns may also affect dosing. Target peak and trough levels for gentamicin, tobramycin, and netilmicin are 6 to 8 μg/ml, and 1 to 2 μg/ml, respectively; for kanamycin and amikacin, 25 to 35 μg/ml and 4 μg/ml, respectively.

Aminoglycosides are inactivated by many β-lactam antibiotics due to formation of a covalent bond between the carboxyl group of a broken β-lactam ring and an amino group of the aminoglycoside. This is clinically important when high doses of a β-lactam are used, as in the case of carbenicillin or ticarcillin.

Adverse Effects

Nephrotoxicity
Ototoxicity
Neuromuscular paralysis is rare

Nephrotoxicity occurs in 5 to 25% of patients. Monitoring serum creatinine is the most useful way to detect nephrotoxicity. Since renal toxicity is usually reversible, alteration of dose with rising serum creatinine is effective.

Ototoxicity, either vestibular or auditory, is a property of all aminoglycosides. It is frequently irreversible, may occur after discontinuing the drug, and may be cumulative with repeated courses of the drug. Not common, auditory toxicity occurs in 0.5 to 3.0% of patients treated; the incidence of vestibular toxicity is 0.4%. Risk factors include duration of aminoglycoside use, elevated blood level, presence of bacteremia, fever, liver dysfunction, use of ethacrynic acid, and the ratio of serum urea nitrogen to serum creatinine as a measure of hypovolemia.

Spectinomycin

A related aminocyclitol (but not an aminoglycoside), spectinomycin is highly active against *N. gonorrhoeae* but not against most other sexually transmitted pathogens.

Tetracyclines and Chloramphenicol

Tetracyclines

Classification of Tetracyclines	
Short acting	Oxytetracycline Tetracycline HCl
Intermediate	Methacycline Demeclocycline
Long acting	Doxycycline Minocycline

Antimicrobial Activity

The antimicrobial spectrums of all tetracyclines are nearly identical. Although broadly active against gram-positive cocci and *E. coli*, many strains, especially those acquired in the hospital, may be resistant. Gonococci and meningococci are very sensitive, but resistant strains of gonococci are common. *Pseudomonas pseudomallei, Brucella* sp., *Vibrio cholerae, Vibrio vulnificus,* and *Mycobacterium marinum* are also sensitive. Spirochetes such as *Borrelia burgdorferi*, rickettsia, chlamydiae, and mycoplasmas are susceptible.

Resistance

Preventing penetration of tetracycline into the bacterial cell is the major mechanism of resistance. Such resistance may be mediated by plasmids.

Pharmacology

Tetracyclines are well-absorbed with peak serum levels occurring in 1 to 3 hours. Absorption is limited by food and by calcium, magnesium, and aluminum in antacids, milk, or iron or iron-containing tonics. They are widely distributed in body fluids and are excreted by the kidney. Dosing intervals are 4 to 8 hours for short acting, 12 hours for intermediate acting, and 12 to 24 hours for long acting.

Adverse Effects

Hypersensitivity reactions are not common
  Anaphylaxis
  Urticaria
  Periorbital edema
  Morbilliform rashes
  Photosensitivity - especially demeclocycline
Teeth and bones
  Discoloration - children < 8 years of age
  Hypoplasia of the enamel - children < 8 years of age
  Depression of skeletal growth - premature infant
Gastrointestinal symptoms
Renal function
  Aggravation of pre-existing renal failure
Nervous and sensory system
  Vertigo - minocycline
Superinfection
  Candida vaginitis
  Thrush

Chloramphenicol

Another product of a *Streptomyces* sp., chloramphenicol inhibits bacterial protein synthesis by reversibly binding to the larger 50S subunit of the 70S ribosome which prevents formation of peptide bonds. It is active against many bacteria, spirochetes, rickettsia, chlamydiae, and mycoplasmas. Salmonellae, including *S. typhi*, are generally susceptible. *H. influenzae, S. pneumoniae,* and *N. meningitidis* are sensitive, but rare instances of resistance are encountered. It is very active against anaerobic bacteria, including *B. fragilis.*

Bacteria become resistant to chloramphenicol by becoming impermeable to the drug, or by producing an enzyme that acetylates the antibiotic to an inactive form.

Chloramphenicol is well-absorbed in the gastrointestinal tract, achieving peak concentrations in 1 hour, and can be give intravenously as well. It is conjugated with glucuronic acid in the liver to an inactive form which is excreted by the kidney. Dosage reduction is required in patients with hyperbilirubinemia.

Chloramphenicol is widely distributed, and it penetrates the blood-brain barrier into the CSF especially well.

Adverse Effects

Hematologic
>Reversible bone marrow depression in adults receiving 4 g or more per day
>Aplastic anemia - 1:24,000 to 40,000 (oral drug only)

Gray baby syndrome in premature infants

Optic neuritis

Rifamycins

Rifampin is a semi-synthetic derivative of a macrocyclic antibiotic compound produced by a *Streptomyces* sp.

It exerts its antibacterial activity by inhibition of DNA-dependent RNA polymerase, which prevents chain initiation.

Rifampin is active against a wide range of micro-organisms. It is extremely active against *S. aureus* and *S. epidermidis*; however, *N. meningitidis*, *N. gonorrhoeae*, and *H. influenzae* are the most sensitive gram-negative specifics. It is active against *Legionella* sp., *Clostridium difficile,* and several *Mycobacterium* sp., including *M. tuberculosis*, *M. ulcerans*, *M. avium-intracellulare* complex, and *M. fortuitum.*

Bacteria rapidly develop resistance due to mutations of β-subunit of the DNA-dependent RNA polymerase.

Rifampin is well-absorbed from the gastrointestinal tract, achieving peak levels 1 to 4 hours after injection. Intravenous rifampin is now available. The half-life is sufficiently long and allows doses to be given only once a day. Rifampin penetrates well into all body tissues and fluids. Staining of contact lenses may occur.

Interaction with many other drugs occur. Rifampin competitively inhibits the hepatic uptake of several compounds. It is a potent inducing agent for hepatic microsomal enzymes, thus leading to shortened half-lives for a number of agents.

Rifabutin (Ansamycin) is an investigational rifamycin S derivative that has been used for *Mycobacterium avium-intracellulare* infection.

Medications for which the Half-Life is Reduced through Enhancement of Hepatic Metabolism by Rifampin

---

Barbituates	Metaprolol
Chloramphenicol	Methadone
Cimetidine	Phenytoin
Clofibrate	Prednisone
Contraceptives, oral	Propranolol
Cyclosporine	Quinidine
Dapsone	Sulfonylureas
Digitoxin	Theophylline
Digoxin	Thyroxine
Estrogens	Verapamil
Itraconazole	Warfarin
Ketoconazole	

Metronidazole

Metronidazole is a very potent and effective agent against anaerobic bacteria, with the exception of nonsporulating gram-positive bacilli and some *Capnocytophaga* sp. It has little activity against other bacteria. Metronidazole is reduced intracellularly and the reduction products are toxic to bacterial cells by interaction with DNA or other macromolecules. The drug is well-absorbed so that oral and IV doses achieve equivalent blood levels. It is distributed widely, including cerebrospinal fluid.

Adverse Effects

Major - rare
   Seizures, encephalopathy
   Cerebellar dysfunction, ataxia
   Peripheral neuropathy
   Disulfiram reaction with alcohol
   Potentiation of effects of warfarin
   Pseudomembranous colitis
   Pancreatitis

Minor
>   Gastrointestinal disturbances
>   Reversible neutropenia
>   Metallic taste
>   Dark or red-brown urine
>   Maculopapular rash, urticaria
>   Urethral, vaginal burning
>   Gynecomastia

Macrolides: Erythromycin and Clindamycin

Erythromycin

Erythromycin is a bacteriostatic macrolide antibiotic.

Erythromycin inhibits RNA-dependent protein synthesis by reversibly binding to the 50S ribosome and preventing chain elongation. Antimicrobial activity is broad against gram-positive and a few gram-negative bacteria, including treponemes, mycoplasmas, chlamydia, and rickettsia. Clinically, the most important organisms inhibited include *S. pneumoniae*, *S. pyogenes*, *C. diphtheriae*, *B. pertussis*, *L. pneumophila*, *M. pneumoniae*, *C. trachomatis*, and *C. pneumoniae*.

Erythromycin is moderately well-absorbed with peak levels occurring in 2 to 4 hours. The base is destroyed by gastric acid, hence the various acid-resistant coatings. Intravenous preparations result in considerably higher blood levels. Erythromycin is distributed through total body water, including middle ear, maxillary sinuses, tonsils, and prostate, but insufficient concentrations are present in CSF to treat meningitis.

Resistance

>   Decreased permeability of the bacterial cell envelope
>   Alteration of the 50S ribosomal receptor site
>   Alteration in the 23S ribosomal RNA by methylation of adenine
>   Inactivation by enzymatic hydrolysis

Adverse Effects

Common
>   Gastrointestinal complaints include cramps, nausea, vomiting, diarrhea

List of Preparations

Preparation	Form	Trade Names
Enteric coated preparations of erythromycin base	Tablets	Ilotycin E-mycin Ery-Tab Robimycin
	Pellets in capsules	Eryc
	Film coated	Filmtab
Stearate salt	Film coated	Erythrocin Bristamycin
Ethylsuccinate ester		Erythrocin Eryped EES Pediamycin
Estolate		Ilosone
Intravenous preparations	Erythromycin gluceptate Erythromycin lactobionate	Ilotycin gluceptate Erythrocin lactobionate

Thrombophlebitis with IV form
Transient hearing loss
Rare
Allergic reactions include skin rash, fever, eosinophilia
Cholestatic hepatitis (estolate)

Clindamycin

Clindamycin binds to 50S ribosome and interferes with chain elongation. It is active against gram-positive cocci such as staphylococci, pneumococci, *S. pyogenes*, and "viridans" streptococci, and against most anaerobes including *B. fragilis*.

Clindamycin is well-absorbed (~ 90%) following oral dosing with peak levels at 1 hour. Higher levels are achieved by IM or IV dosing. There is good penetration of most tissue except the CSF. The half-life is such that doses must be repeated at 4- to 6-hour intervals.

Adverse Effects

Allergic reactions
  Rash, fever, erythema multiforme, anaphylaxis
Diarrhea
  "Toxic" (common)
  C. difficile pseudomembranous colitis (less common)
Hepatotoxicity
  Aminotransferase elevation
Reversible neutropenia, thrombocytopenia, agranulocytosis

Vancomycin

Vancomycin inhibits synthesis and assembly of the second stage of cell wall peptidoglycan polymers. Its effects are bactericidal, and development of resistance is rare.

Vancomycin is active against S. aureus and S. epidermidis, including strains resistant to methicillin. S. pyogenes, other streptococci, pneumococci, enterococci, corynebacteria JK, and Clostridium difficile are sensitive. Vancomycin is only effective against systemic infection if given intravenously. The oral nonabsorbable form is effective against C. difficile.

Target peak serum levels are 30 to 40 µg/ml; trough levels should be 5 to 10 µg/ml.

Adverse Effects

Fever, chills, phlebitis
"Red man syndrome" (seen with rapid IV administration)
Rash
Reversible leukopenia or eosinophilia
Neurotoxicity
  Hearing loss is infrequent if serum concentration < 40 µg/ml
  Tinnitus

Sulfonamides

Sulfonamides are bacteriostatic chemical entities that competitively inhibit the incorporation of p-aminobenzoic acid (PABA) into tetrahydropteroic acid, thus inhibiting folic acid synthesis.

Classification of Sulfonamides

Short acting	Sulfisoxazole
	Sulfamethoxazole
	Sulfadiazine
	Sulfamethizole
Long acting	Sulfadoxine
Limited to gastrointestinal tract	Sulfaguanidine
	Sulfasuxidine
	Sulfathalidine
	Salicylazosulfapyridine
Topical	Mafenide acetate
	Silver sulfadiazine

Sulfonamides are active against a broad spectrum of gram-negative and gram-positive bacteria, as well as *Actinomyces, Chlamydia, Plasmodia,* and *Toxoplasma.* Resistance is common and limits the usefulness of the sulfonamides.

Sulfonamides are well-absorbed from the gastrointestinal tract and well-distributed throughout blood fluids, including CSF. They are metabolized by acetylation and glucuronidation in the liver, and metabolized products appear in the urine.

Adverse Effects

Nausea, vomiting, diarrhea
Rash

Fever
Headache
Depression
Jaundice, hepatic necrosis
Serum sickness-like syndrome
Acute hemolytic anemia
Agranulocytosis, thrombocytopenia, leukopenia
Increased warfarin activity by displacement from albumin binding sites

Trimethoprim

Trimethoprim is a dihydrofolate reductase inhibitor that potentiates the activity of sulfonamides by sequential inhibition of folic acid synthesis. It is active against many gram-positive cocci and most gram-negative rods except *Pseudomonas aeruginosa* and *Bacteroides* sp.

The combination of trimethoprim-sulfamethoxazole (cotrimoxazole) is active against *S. aureus, S. pyogenes, S. pneumoniae, E. coli, Proteus mirabilis, Shigella* sp., *Salmonella* sp., *Pseudomonas cepacia, Pseudomonas pseudomallei, Yersinia enterocolitica,* and *N. gonorrhoeae.* It is clinically active against *Pneumocystis carinii.*

Trimethoprim resistance is most commonly due to plasmid-mediated changes in dihydrofolate reductase.

Trimethoprim is very well-absorbed from the gastrointestinal tract, and it is distributed in most body fluids. It is concentrated two- to threefold in prostatic fluid compared to serum. It is excreted unchanged by the kidney via tubular secretion.

Adverse Effects

Nausea, vomiting, diarrhea, anorexia
Hypersensitivity reactions
　　Rash
Impaired folate utilization
　　Megaloblastic marrow
Leukopenia, thrombocytopenia, granulocytopenia
Pseudomembranous colitis

Quinolones

The quinolones inhibit DNA synthesis in bacterial cells, but not mammalian cells, by inhibition of DNA topoisomerases (gyrases).

Nalidixic acid is active against gram-negative rods and, to a lesser extent, gram-positive bacteria. The newer quinolones are considerably ($\geq$ 100-fold) more active and the spectrum is expanded. Activity against gram-positive cocci is less than versus gram-negative cocci. Activity against anaerobes is poor.

Resistance

Most resistance is due to one of two mechanisms: (1) mutations in the gene coding for DNA gyrase, and (2) mutations that change the outer membrane porins.

Pharmacology

The quinolones are well-absorbed from the gastrointestinal tract, with peaks occurring 1 to 2 hours after administration. Absorption is delayed by food and is reduced by magnesium, aluminum or calcium antacids and by sucralfate and iron salts.

Adverse Effects

Gastrointestinal side-effects
Central nervous system side-effects
    Mild: headache, dizziness, tiredness, insomnia, faintness, agitation, listlessness, restlessness, abnormal vision, bad dreams
    Severe: hallucinations, depression, psychotic reactions, grand mal convulsions
    Skin and allergic reactions
    Erythema urticaria, rash, pruritus, photosensitivity reactions
Drug interactions (varies with quinolone)
    False positive urine test for glucose with Benedict solution (Clinitest)
    Enhanced effects of theophylline
    Interference with clearance of caffeine and theophylline
    Probenecid raises blood levels
Arthropathy in immature animals receiving some quinolones has prompted caution in using this class of agent in children

In Vitro Activity of Selected 4-Quinolones

	Nalidixic Acid	Ciprofloxacin	Enoxacin	Norfloxacin	Ofloxacin	Pefloxacin
Gram negative aerobes						
E. coli	+	+++	++	+++	+++	+++
K. pneumoniae	+	+++	++	+++	+++	+++
Enterobacter	—	+++	++	++	++	++
S. marcescens	—	++	+	++	++	++
Salmonella	—	+++	++	+++	+++	+++
Pseudomonas	—	++	+	+	+	+
H. influenzae	+	+++	+++	+++	+++	+++
Gram positive aerobes						
S. aureus (methicillin sensitive and methicillin resistant[a])	—	++	+	+	++	++
S. pyogenes	—	+	—	—	—	—
Enterococcus	—	+	—	—	+	—
Anaerobes						
B. fragilis	—	—	—	—	—	—
Gram positive cocci	—	—	—	—	—	—

+, some activity; ++, moderate activity; +++, great activity; —, little or no activity.
[a]Resistance may develop rapidly in methicillin resistant isolates.

Antimycobacterial Agents

Drugs	Mechanism of Action	Selected Pharmacologic Properties	Adverse Effects
First line drugs			
Isoniazid	Inhibits synthesis of mycolic acid	Oral or IM CSF levels 20% of plasma Metabolism by acetylation in liver Slow acetylators (5-83% of different populations) Rapid acetylators No dosage modification in moderate hepatic or renal failure, but reduction in dosage necessary in severe renal failure	Elevated ALT Hepatitis (rare <20 yr; 2.3% >50 yr) Peripheral neuropathy Psychosis Hypersensitivity reactions Others - rare Dupuytren's contractions Shoulder-hand syndrome Pellagra Pyridoxine deficiency - related anemia Drug interactions: Phenytoin toxicity potentiated
Ethambutol	Affects RNA synthesis	Oral only Good CSF penetration with inflammation Renal excretion; modify dose in renal failure	Retrobulbar neuritis Impairment of visual acuity or color vision Gastrointestinal symptoms Hyperuricemia Hypersensitivity - dermatitis, arthralgia, fever
Rifampin	Inhibits DNA dependent RNA polymerase	Oral and IV Widely distributed, including CSF Deacetylated: biliary excretion and enterohepatic recirculation Excretion primarily into gastrointestinal tract Modify dose for liver but not renal failure	Hepatotoxicity Alcoholics prone to serious toxicity Hypersensitivity reactions Flushing Fever Pruritus Eosinophilia Hemolysis

Antimycobacterial Agents *(Continued)*

Drugs	Mechanism of Action	Selected Pharmacologic Properties	Adverse Effects
			Interstitial nephritis
			Flu-like syndrome
			Orange color in body fluids
			Induces P-450 liver enzymes
			Increases metabolism of ketoconazole, cyclosporine, digoxin, phenytoin, prednisone, itraconazole, propanolol, and other drugs
Streptomycin	Inhibits protein synthesis Binds to 50S ribosome	An aminoglycoside	Renal toxicity Ototoxicity
Pyrazinamide	Unknown	Oral only Widely distributed Crosses inflamed meninges	Hepatotoxicity
Second line drugs			
Amithiozone (thiacetazone)	Unknown	Oral Low price Twice weekly administration	Gastrointestinal toxicity Bone marrow suppression
Para-amino-salicylic acid	Inhibits folate synthesis	Oral only Incompletely absorbed	Gastrointestinal intolerance Reversible lupus-like syndrome Mononucleosis-like syndrome Hypersensitivity reactions frequent
Cycloserine	Inhibits cell wall synthesis	Oral Well absorbed and widely distributed	Peripheral neuropathy CNS dysfunction Seizures

Ethionamide	Unknown	Well absorbed Widely distributed, including CSF	Gastrointestinal irritation Nausea, vomiting Peripheral neuropathy Psychiatric disturbances Hepatotoxicity
Kanamycin	Unknown	An aminoglycoside	Ototoxicity Nephrotoxicity
Viomycin	Unknown; complex boric polypeptide		Ototoxicity Nephrotoxicity
Capreomycin	Unknown; polypeptide		Ototoxicity Nephrotoxicity
Amikacin	Unknown	An aminoglycoside	Ototoxicity Nephrotoxicity
Rifabutin	Inhibits DNA dependent RNA polymerase	Oral Long half-life High tissue concentrations	Hepatotoxicity Alcoholics prone to serious toxicity Hypersensitivity reactions Flushing Fever Pruritus Eosinophilia Hemolysis Interstitial nephritis Flu-like syndrome Orange color in body fluids Induces P-450 liver enzymes Increases metabolism of ketoconazole, cyclosporine, digoxin, phenytoin, prednisone, itraconazole, propanolol, and other drugs

(Continues)

Antimycobacterial Agents *(Continued)*

Drugs	Mechanism of Action	Selected Pharmacologic Properties	Adverse Effects
Drugs for treatment of leprosy			
Dapsone (DDS)	Interferes with folate synthesis A sulfone	Oral Well absorbed Acetylated, renal excretion Modify dose in renal failure	Minor hemolysis Methemoglobinemia
Acedapsone	A sulfone	Long-acting form of dapsone	
Sulfoxone	A sulfone		
Rifampin		(See listing under first line drugs, above)	
Clofazimine	Unknown	Absorption variable Widely distributed in reticuloendothelial tissues Not metabolized Excreted slowly - biliary route	Gastrointestinal intolerance Skin pigmentations

Antifungal Agents

Drugs	Mechanism of Action	Selected Pharmacologic Properties	Adverse Effects
Amphotericin B	Combines with sterols in fungal cytoplasmic membrane	IV only - desoxycholate formulation Colloidal solution Drug is bound to cholesterol containing membranes and β-lipoproteins. Stored in liver and other organs Degraded in situ; not excreted in bile or urine	Fever, rigors Hypoxemia, hypotension, or hypertension Azotemia - very common Headache Phlebitis Thrombocytopenia, leukopenia - rare Anaphylaxis - rare Burning sensation of soles of feet - rare
Clotrimazole	Decreases ergosterol synthesis	Topical	Local irritation
Fluconazole	Decreases ergosterol synthesis	Oral or IV Completely absorbed from gastrointestinal tract; not dependent on acid Excreted unchanged in urine Penetration into body fluids including CSF excellent (levels 70% of serum)	Gastrointestinal toxicity
Flucytosine (5-FC)	Interferes with DNA synthesis	Oral Absorption rapid and complete Widely distributed including CSF Excreted by kidney (90%) Half-life short, requiring q6h dosing	Rash Diarrhea Hepatic dysfunction In patients with azotemia or those also receiving amphotericin B: Leukopenia Thrombocytopenia Enterocolitis

(Continues)

Antifungal Agents *(Continued)*

Drugs	Mechanism of Action	Selected Pharmacologic Properties	Adverse Effects
Griseofulvin		Oral Metabolized in liver Long half-life	Headache
Itraconazole	Decreases ergosterol synthesis	Oral Absorption good Distribution to tissues good, but not to CSF	Nausea
Ketoconazole	Decreases ergosterol synthesis	Oral only Absorption good, but reduced by H₂ receptor blockers Metabolized by liver, excreted as inactive drug in bile and urine Blood levels lowered by rifampin Poor penetration into CSF, saliva, breast milk, vaginal secretions	Anorexia Nausea Vomiting Rash, pruritus Reduced serum testosterone Reduced response to ACTH Hepatitis - rare Hypertension - rare With prolonged therapy: Gynecomastia Impotence Decreased libido Oligospermia Azoospermia Menstrual irregularities
Miconazole	Decreases ergosterol synthesis	Topical IV	Local irritation
Nystatin	Similar to amphotericin B	Oral Topical Poorly absorbed	

Antiviral Agents

Drugs	Mechanism of Action	Selected Pharmacologic Properties	Adverse Effects
Acyclovir	Phosphorylated by HSV induced thymidine kinase Inhibits viral polymerases	Oral and IV use Oral bioavailability low Peak concentrations 1.5 hours after oral dosing Volume of distribution corresponds to total body water CSF levels ½ blood levels Half-life short, 4-hour dosing common Excreted mostly unmetabolized by kidney	Renal dysfunction - 5% Reversible Neurotoxicity - 1% Lethargy Obtundation Tremors Hallucinations Delirium Seizures Coma Gastrointestinal toxicity with oral
Amantadine	Blocks uncoating of viral genome in lysosomes	Oral only Well absorbed; peak levels 2-4 hours after dosing Widely distributed, including CSF Blood levels 2 times in elderly vs. young adults for same dose Excreted unmetabolized by kidney	Minor gastrointestinal toxicity CNS complaints Nervousness Lightheadedness Difficulty concentrating Insomnia Loss of appetite
Didanosine (dideoxy-inosine [ddI])	Inhibition of reverse transcriptase	Oral only Half-life 1.6 hours Bioavailability 40%	Diarrhea - common Painful peripheral neuropathy - common Lower extremities Major dose limiting toxicity Pancreatitis (1.5-2.0% of patients) Electrolyte abnormalities - hypokalemia, hypocalcemia, hypomagnesemia, increased serum uric acid Rare - liver enzyme elevation Rash, thrombocytopenia, neutropenia

(Continues)

Antiviral Agents *(Continued)*

Drugs	Mechanism of Action	Selected Pharmacologic Properties	Adverse Effects
Dideoxycytidine (ddC) (see Zalcitabine)			
Foscarnet	Inhibits herpesvirus DNA polymerase and HIV reverse transcriptase	IV Penetrates CSF, eye Requires IV hydration	Nephrotoxicity in one-third of patients Vomiting Hypocalcemia, hypomagnesemia, hypophosphatemia Seizures
Ganciclovir	Phosphorylated by infection induced kinases Triphosphate form inhibits viral DNA polymerase	IV only Oral bioavailability very low Short half-life requires q4-6h dosing Excreted unmetabolized by kidney (> 90%)	Leukopenia (47% of patients) Neutropenia Thrombocytopenia CNS side-effects (5-15% of patients): Headache Behavioral changes Psychosis Convulsions Coma Anemia Rash Fever Liver function test abnormalities Thrombophlebitis at infusion site
Idoxuridine	Triphosphate inhibits viral DNA synthesis Incorporated in viral and cellular DNA	Topical use (ophthalmic) only	Pain Pruritus Inflammation Edema
Interferon alfa	Depending on virus and cell type, interferon inhibits: Viral penetration or uncoating Synthesis or methylation of	IV and IM or subcutaneous Local injection Production of a unique protein 2',5'-oligoadenylate synthetase; this is used as a marker of antiviral state Antiviral state begins in 1-6 hours	Influenza-like syndrome Nausea, vomiting, diarrhea Bone marrow suppression Granulocytopenia Thrombocytopenia Neurotoxicity Somnolence

	Mechanism	Pharmacokinetics	Adverse effects
	messenger RNA Translation of viral proteins Viral assembly and release	and lasts 1-6 days depending on cell system Clearance is by inactivation by body fluids and metabolism	Confusion Behavioral disturbance EEG changes Reversible neurasthenia Anorexia, weight loss Myalgia with prolonged therapy Elevation of hepatic enzymes Elevated triglyceride levels Renal insufficiency Local reaction
Ribavirin	Multiple effects on DNA and RNA viruses except single-stranded RNA viruses Inhibits IMPDH and interferes with GTP synthesis Inhibits influenza virus RNA polymerase	Aerosol Oral Oral bioavailability is 45% Peak plasma concentrations 1-2 hours Widely distributed including CSF (% of plasma levels) Elimination is complex because of active metabolites Accumulation occurs during chronic administration Aerosol administration results in very high respiratory secretion levels *and* significant blood levels	Anemia, macrocytic, dose dependent due to extravascular hemolysis and, at higher doses, bone marrow suppression Increased reticulocyte counts when oral treatment is stopped Increases of serum bilirubin, serum iron, and uric acid - reversible Gastrointestinal toxicity - mild CNS complaints Headache Lethargy Insomnia Mood alteration Aerosol: Conjunctival irritation - mild Rash Wheezing - transient Deterioration in pulmonary function - reversible
Trifluridine	Triphosphate competes with deoxythymidine triphosphate Incorporated into DNA Inhibits viral DNA synthesis	Topical (ophthalmic) only	Discomfort Palpebral edema Irritation Superficial punctate keratopathy

(Continues)

Antiviral Agents *(Continued)*

Drugs	Mechanism of Action	Selected Pharmacologic Properties	Adverse Effects
Vidarabine	Triphosphate competitively inhibits viral DNA polymerase Incorporated into DNA Inhibits other enzymes Result is inhibition of viral DNA synthesis	Topical (ophthalmic) IV Rapidly deaminated to hypoxanthine arabinoside by adenosine deaminase Infused over 12-24 hours Primary route of clearance is renal Poor solubility requires large fluid volumes for infusion	Gastrointestinal toxicity Anorexia Nausea Vomiting Diarrhea Weight loss Thrombophlebitis at infusion site Weakness Hypokalemia Rash Inappropriate secretion of ADH
Zalcitabine (Dideoxycytidine, ddC)	Inhibition of reverse transcriptase	Oral only Well absorbed Half-life 1-2 hours Oral bioavailability 60-90% Low CSF penetration	Peripheral neuropathy - common Low extremities Dose related and dose limiting Maculovesicular eruptions Aphthous oral ulcerations Fever
Zidovudine (AZT, azido-thymidine)	Inhibition of viral RNA-dependent DNA polymerase (reverse transcriptase)	Oral only Oral bioavailability is 60-65% Rapidly absorbed; peak concentration in ½ to 1½ hours Widely distributed including CSF Rapidly metabolized Renal clearance of zidovudine and metabolite Must be administered frequently (q4h)	Granulocytopenia Anemia - 45% of patients Headache Nausea Insomnia Myalgia Neurotoxicity Seizures Wernicke's encephalopathy Polymyositis Muscle wasting Nail pigmentation Drugs that inhibit glucuronidation and/or renal excretion increase marrow toxicity

Antiparasitic Agents

Drugs	Selected Pharmacologic Properties	Major Adverse Effects
Albendazole	Oral only Not well absorbed Metabolized in the liver	Well tolerated in single dose regimens High dose, prolonged therapy Hepatitis, obstructive jaundice
Amphotericin B	See Antifungals	See Antifungals
Bithionol	Oral	Urticaria Photosensitivity reaction Gastrointestinal complaints
Chloroquine	Oral; IV Rapidly absorbed, slowly excreted Widely distributed 50% excreted in urine, 50% metabolized Long half-life allows once a week dosing Concentrated in erythrocytes IV administration must be given slowly and with great caution to avoid cardiovascular collapse and/or seizures	Occasional temporary side-effects Headache, nausea, vomiting Blurred vision, dizziness Fatigue, confusion Rare - depigmentation Irreversible retinopathy (doses >250 mg daily) Corneal opacities Weight loss, leukopenia Myalgias Exacerbation of skin diseases
Diethylcarbamazine	Oral only Well absorbed, well distributed Short half-life Excreted via kidney	Headache Malaise Weakness Systemic reactions due to release of filarial antigen
Diloxanide furoate	Oral only Excreted in urine Low cost	Mild gastrointestinal complaints

(Continues)

Antiparasitic Agents *(Continued)*

Drugs	Selected Pharmacologic Properties	Major Adverse Effects
Iodoquinol	Oral only Best tolerated with meals	Headache Gastrointestinal complaints Iodine dermatitis - occasional
Ivermectin	Oral or parenteral Excreted in stool Concentrated in liver and adipose tissue	Well tolerated Initiation of treatment may cause transient fever, pruritus, headache, cutaneous edema
Macrolide antibiotics Clindamycin Spiramycin	See Macrolides - Antibacterials	See Macrolides - Antibacterials
Mebendazole	Oral only Poorly absorbed from gastrointestinal tract Metabolized, then renally excreted	Few side effects at low doses Transient abdominal pain and diarrhea High doses Alopecia, liver enzyme abnormalities Transient bone marrow suppression
Mefloquine	Oral only Incompletely absorbed, widely distributed Extensively metabolized Long half-life	Generally well-tolerated Sinus bradycardia 7% Seizures
Melarsoprol B	An arsenical IV only	Highly toxic Encephalopathy - results in mortality in 6% of recipients Fever, hypertension, abdominal pain, vomiting, arthralgia
Metronidazole	See Metronidazole - Antibacterials	See Metronidazole - Antibacterials

Drug	Pharmacokinetics	Toxicity/Side Effects
Niclosamide	Oral Poorly absorbed	Very well tolerated Occasional mild gastrointestinal symptoms Lightheadedness Rash
Nifurtimox	Oral Well absorbed	Toxicity - 40-70% of patients Gastrointestinal - nausea, vomiting, abdominal pain, anorexia, weight loss Neurologic - restlessness, disorientation, insomnia, twitching, paresthesias, polyneuritis, weakness, stiffness
Oxamniquine	Oral Excreted by kidney	Dizziness - 40% of patients Drowsiness Convulsions Red color to urine
Paromomycin	See Aminoglycosides - Antibacterials	See Aminoglycosides - Antibacterials
Pentamidine isethionate	IM, IV, aerosol Highly tissue bound Excreted slowly Does not penetrate CNS	IM - local reactions, hypotension IV - cardiac arrhythmias, nausea, vomiting, dizziness, rash, facial flushing Breathlessness Metallic taste Hypotension Hypoglycemia - 6-9% of patients Diabetes mellitus Reversible renal failure - 25% Leukopenia, thrombocytopenia, elevated transaminase Fever Hypocalcemia Confusion Hallucinations Aerosolized - much better tolerated Bronchospasm Pharyngeal irritation Metallic taste

(Continues)

Antiparasitic Agents *(Continued)*

Drugs	Selected Pharmacologic Properties	Major Adverse Effects
Praziquantel	Oral only Partially absorbed Excreted by kidney Long half-life	Generally well tolerated Reactions common but mild and transient Nausea, vomiting, abdominal pain Dizziness, headache, lassitude
Primaquine	Oral Well absorbed	Hemolysis in G6PD deficiency Gastrointestinal complaints
Proguanil	Oral only Slowly absorbed Daily dose required	High doses - gastrointestinal symptoms
Pyrantel pamoate	Oral only Poorly absorbed	Minimal toxicity Gastrointestinal symptoms Headache Dizziness
Pyrimethamine/short-acting sulfonamides	Sulfadiazine or trisulfapyrimidines usually used Pyrimethamine is well absorbed Extensively metabolized Half-life 4-6 days	Pyrimethamine Well tolerated Rare - blood dyscrasias, rash, vomiting, seizures, shock Bone marrow suppression with higher doses Sulfonamides Allergic reactions Gastrointestinal complaints AIDS patients - 60% have untoward effect to combinations: fever, rash, bone marrow suppression, hepatotoxicity

Pyrimethamine-sulfadoxine (Fansidar)	Well absorbed Sulfadoxine half-life 5-9 days	Rare severe reactions due to sulfadoxine Cutaneous including toxic epidermal necrolysis, erythema multiforme, Stevens-Johnson syndrome Other side-effects - rare Serum sickness Bone marrow suppression Hepatitis Hepatic granuloma Pneumonitis
Quinacrine	Oral only Well absorbed, widely distributed	Bitter taste Nausea, vomiting Headache, dizziness Yellow skin - high doses (4% of patients treated) Rare - psychosis Drug interactions Disulfiram-like effect Interferes with metabolism of primaquine
Quinidine	IV	ECG changes
Quinine	Oral Well absorbed Metabolized by liver, excreted in urine	Cinchonism - tinnitus, decreased hearing, headache, dysphoria, nausea, vomiting, visual disturbances Dose related and reversible Uncommon - rash, angioedema of face, pruritus, agranulocytosis Respiratory depression in patients with myasthenia gravis Hypoglycemia in patients with high *Pl. falciparum* parasitemia

(Continues)

Antiparasitic Agents *(Continued)*

Drugs	Selected Pharmacologic Properties	Major Adverse Effects
Stibogluconate sodium	Parenteral Long half-life Renal excretion	Relatively well-tolerated Abdominal pain Nausea, vomiting, malaise Headache
Suramin	Parenteral only Long half-life Negligible metabolism Does not penetrate CNS	Immediate - nausea, vomiting, shock, loss of consciousness, fever, urticaria Late - fever, rash, exfoliative dermatitis Stomatitis Paresthesias of the palms and soles
Tetracyclines Tetracycline Doxycycline	See Tetracyclines - Antibacterials	See Tetracyclines - Antibacterials
Thiabendazole	Oral only Rapidly absorbed Excreted or metabolized in urine	50% of patients experience side effects Most common - nausea, anorexia, vomiting, dizziness Less common - diarrhea, epigastric pain, pruritus, drowsiness, giddiness, headache

Section 2

EMPIRIC THERAPY FOR INFECTIOUS SYNDROMES

Syndrome	Likely Disease or Pathogen	Therapy	Comment
		FEVER	
Acute severe illness with fever and rash	Meningococcemia Rocky Mountain Spotted Fever Toxic shock Acute endocarditis	Cefotaxime or Ceftriaxone Both + chloramphenicol	Rash of toxic shock, "sunburn-like," others macular to petechial
		UPPER RESPIRATORY INFECTIONS	
Pharyngitis	S. pyogenes (group A)	Penicillin or Erythromycin	10 days of therapy needed to prevent sequelae, consider other causes
Otitis externa	Staph aureus, S. pyogenes P. aeruginosa, Proteus sp.	Cloxacillin or Amoxicillin-clavulanate or Trimethoprim-sulfamethoxazole	Irrigation to remove cerumen may be helpful, mild cases may be treated topically, gram-negative rods usually do not require treatment
Otitis externa— malignant	Staph aureus, P. aeruginosa (especially diabetics)	Ticarcillin-clavulanate or Imipenem or Both + gentamicin or Ciprofloxacin	
Otitis media and mastoiditis	S. pneumoniae, H. influenzae M. catarrhalis	Amoxicillin-clavulanate or Cefuroxime axetil or Trimethoprim-sulfamethoxazole or Cefuroxime or Cefotaxime/ceftriaxone/ceftizoxime	Chronic may be due to Staph or enteric gram-negatives

Sinusitis–acute	S. pneumoniae, H. influenzae	Amoxicillin–clavulanate or Cefuroxime axetil or Trimethoprim-sulfamethoxazole or Clarithromycin	Nasal decongestants help drainage
Sinusitis–chronic	Above plus anaerobes, Staph aureus, gram-negative rods	Amoxicillin–clavulanate or Cefuroxime axetil + metronidazole	Use Gram stain and culture as guide, may need surgical drainage
Epiglottitis	H. influenzae	Cefotaxime/ceftriaxone/ceftizoxime or Chloramphenicol	Maintain adequate airway
Odontogenic infection	Aerobic and anaerobic streptococci, fusobacteria, Bacteroides	Amoxicillin–clavulanate or Ampicillin-sulbactam or Clindamycin or Penicillin + metronidazole	Surgical drainage may be necessary
Acute parotitis	Staph aureus Mumps virus	Nafcillin/oxacillin or Vancomycin	Express pus from duct
Suppurative thyroiditis	Staph aureus, S. pyogenes S. pneumoniae	Nafcillin/oxacillin or Vancomycin	
Acute bronchitis (no chronic bronchitis)	Viral, Mycoplasma pneumoniae, S. pneumoniae, H. influenzae, Chlamydia pneumoniae	Symptomatic or Erythromycin or Doxycycline or Amoxicillin–clavulanate or Trimethoprim-sulfamethoxazole or Clarithromycin	Value of antibiotic unproven in previously healthy adults

(Continues)

Syndrome	Likely Disease or Pathogen	Therapy	Comment
Acute exacerbation of chronic bronchitis	S. pneumoniae, H. influenzae, M. catarrhalis, M. pneumoniae, C. pneumoniae, viruses	Amoxicillin-clavulanate or Trimethoprim-sulfamethoxazole or Cefuroxime axetil or Doxycycline or Clarithromycin	
LOWER RESPIRATORY INFECTION			
Bronchiolitis	Respiratory syncytial virus	Ribavirin	First 2 yrs of life, administer via respirator
Pneumonia Acute community-acquired	S. pneumoniae, H. influenzae, L. pneumophila, M. pneumoniae, C. pneumoniae, Staph aureus, influenza virus	Cefuroxime or Cefotaxime/ceftriaxone/ceftizoxime or Amoxicillin-clavulanate (Consider addition of erythromycin or clarithromycin)	Gram stain of sputum may be helpful, consider amantadine during influenza A outbreak
"Atypical"	M. pneumonia, L. pneumophila, C. pneumoniae	Erythromycin or Clarithromycin	Younger person, less acute, myalgias, headache
Aspiration (community)	B. melaninogenicus, other Bacteroides, Fusobacterium spp., aerobic and anaerobic streptococci	Clindamycin or Cefoxitin/cefotetan/cefmetazole or Amoxicillin-clavulanate or Ampicillin-sulbactam	Foul sputum, chronicity, hx of aspiration
Aspiration (hospital) and nosocomial	Above + enteric gram-negative rods and Staph aureus	Imipenem or	If pseudomonas is pathogen, add gentamicin

Condition	Pathogens	Therapy	Comments
		Ticarcillin-clavulanate or Ceftazidime + clindamycin or Clindamycin + aztreonam/ciprofloxacin/gentamicin	
Empyema	*Staph. aureus, S. pneumoniae, S. pyogenes*	Nafcillin/oxacillin or Cefazolin or Vancomycin	Drainage essential, usually via chest tube
Lung abscess	See aspiration pneumonia—community and aspiration pneumonia—hospital-acquired	See aspiration pneumonia—community and aspiration pneumonia—hospital-acquired	Rarely requires surgical approach to abscess
Pneumonia, bronchitis, bronchiectasis in cystic fibrosis patients	Community-acquired pathogens plus *Staph. aureus, P. aeruginosa*	Ticarcillin-clavulanate or Piperacillin/mezlocillin/azlocillin/ticarcillin or Ceftazidime or Imipenem or Ciprofloxacin/ofloxacin ± gentamicin for all of above	May respond to therapy that does not cover pseudomonas even if present, amikacin useful if gentamicin resistance common
URINARY TRACT INFECTIONS			
Acute pyelonephritis	*E. coli,* also Proteus, Klebsiella Enterobacter, Enterococci	Cefotaxime/ceftriaxone/cefoperazone/ceftazidime or Trimethoprim/sulfamethoxazole or Ampicillin-sulbactam or Ciprofloxacin/ofloxacin or Piperacillin/mezlocillin/azlocillin/ticarcillin-clavulanate	Evaluate for obstruction, Gram stain of urine is helpful

(Continues)

Syndrome	Likely Disease or Pathogen	Therapy	Comment
Chronic pyelonephritis	As above plus *P. aeruginosa*	As above with or without gentamicin	Gram stain and prior culture results helpful amikacin useful if gentamicin resistance is significant
Cystitis—lower tract infection	*E. coli, Staph saprophyticus, C. trachomatis,* other enteric gram-negative rods, enterococci	Trimethoprim/sulfamethoxazole or Ciprofloxacin/ofloxacin/norfloxacin or Amoxicillin-clavulanate or Cephalexin or Cefuroxime axetil	Consider pelvic examination to document *C. trachomatis*
Prostatitis	Gram-negative enteric organisms, *N. gonorrhoeae, C. trachomatis*	Ofloxacin/ciprofloxacin or Trimethoprin-sulfamethoxazole or Trimethoprim	Duration of 1–3 months often needed
SEPSIS			
(severe systemic illness often with bacteremia)			
general: use parenteral agents, consider anti-endotoxin antibody therapy			
Sepsis—urinary tract source	Gram-negative enteric organisms plus enterococci	Cefotaxime/ceftriaxone/ceftizoxime/cefoperazone/ceftazidime or Piperacillin/mezlocillin/azlocillin/ticarcillin/ticarcillin-clavulanate or Aztreonam or Imipenem or Ciprofloxacin All ± gentamicin	Relieve obstruction, Gram stain may be helpful

Sepsis—skin source	Staphylococci, streptococci	Nafcillin/oxacillin or Cefazolin or Vancomycin	
Sepsis—gut source	Enteric gram-negative rods plus *B. fragilis* and anaerobic cocci	Cefotaxime/ceftriaxone/ceftizoxime/ cefoperazone/ceftazidime All + metronidazole or Ticarcillin/clavulanate or Imipenem or Ampicillin/sulbactam or Clindamycin + gentamicin or Aztreonam + metronidazole or Cefoxitin/cefotetan/cefmetazole + gentamicin	Amikacin useful if gentamicin resistance is common
Sepsis—neutropenic patient	Enteric gram-negative rods (including pseudomonas), staphylococci, viridans streptococci	Ticarcillin/piperacillin/mezlocillin/ azlocillin/ticarcillin-clavulanate All + gentamicin or Ceftazidime/cefoperazone + ticarcillin/piperacillin/ mezlocillin/azlocillin or Imipenem or Ceftazidime	Vancomycin should be added with line sepsis or when resistant gram-positives are suspected, amikacin useful where gentamicin resistance is common

(Continues)

PERITONITIS AND INTRA-ABDOMINAL INFECTION

Syndrome	Likely Disease or Pathogen	Therapy	Comment
Primary peritonitis	Enteric gram-negative rods, S. pneumoniae	Cefotaxime/ceftriaxone/ceftizoxime/ cefoperazone or Ticarcillin/piperacillin/mezlocillin/ azlocillin/ticarcillin-clavulanate All + gentamicin or Imipenem	Seen in patients with ascites
Secondary peritonitis	Enteric gram-negative rods, Bacteroides fragilis, Bacteroides sp., anaerobic cocci	Cefotaxime/ceftriaxone/ ceftizoxime/cefoperazone/ Ceftazidime all + metronidazole or Imipenem or Ticarcillin-clavulanate or Ampicillin-sulbactam or Clindamycin + gentamicin or Aztreonam + metronidazole or Cefoxitin/cefotetan/cefmetazole + gentamicin	Enterococci may be present although initial treatment for this organism is not usually necessary, candida may be seen in impaired hosts and older patients
Intraperitoneal abscess	As above	As above	Usually requires drainage
Peritonitis with continous ambulatory peritoneal dialysis	Coagulase-negative staphylococci enteric gram-negative rods, Staph aureus	Initial dose of vancomycin 1 gram/liter intraperitoneally + gentamicin 60 mg/liter intraperitoneally	Maintenance of vancomycin 25 mg/liter of dialysate plus gentamicin 8 mg/liter dialysate May require systemic therapy
Pancreatic abscess	As above with addition of Staph aureus	Cefotaxime/ceftriaxone/ceftizoxime All + metronidazole or Imipenem	Usually requires drainage

Liver abscess		or Cefoxitin/cefotetan/cefmetazole or Ticarcillin-clavulanate All + gentamicin	As above
Liver abscess	As above but must consider amebic abscess	As above—metronidazole effective for amebic abscess	
Splenic abscess	*Staph aureus*, streptococci, enteric gram-negative rods (including salmonella)	Cefotaxime/ceftriaxone/ceftizoxime or Imipenem	May be seen with endocarditis
Acute appendicitis	See secondary peritonitis	See secondary peritonitis	Surgical therapy usually needed, Yersinia infection may mimic appendicitis
Acute cholecystitis and acute cholangitis	Enteric gram-negative rods, anaerobes including Bacteroides, clostridia, fusobacterium, and enterococci	Cefotaxime/ceftazidime/ Ceftizoxime/cefoperazone All + metronidazole or Imipenem or Ticarcillin-clavulanate or Ampicillin-sulbactam or Cefoxitin/cefotetan/cefmetazole All + gentamicin	

CARDIOVASCULAR INFECTIONS

| Endocarditis on native valve | Viridans streptococci, enterococci, *Staph aureus*, *Staph epidermidis* and HACEK group (Haemophilus, Actinobacillus, Cardiobacterium, Eikenella, Kingella) | Vancomycin + gentamicin + ampicillin
or
Nafcillin + ampicillin/penicillin + gentamicin | Isolation of organism and sensitivity testing extremely valuable |

(Continues)

Syndrome	Likely Disease or Pathogen	Therapy	Comment
Endocarditis on prosthetic valve	Above plus gram-negative aerobes	Ceftazidime + vancomycin + gentamicin	Fungi are a possibility
Endocarditis with "negative" blood cultures	Above plus fastidious streptococci, HACEK group	Ampicillin + vancomycin + gentamicin	Legionella, Brucella, and Chlamydia, Histoplasma and Q fever should be considered
Suppurative thrombophlebitis	Staphylococci (aureus and coagulase-negative), gram-negative enteric rods	Vancomycin + ceftazidime	Gram stain of pus helpful, consider Candida
Vascular graft infection	Staphylococci (aureus and coagulase-negative), streptococci, coagulase-negative enteric rods	Vancomycin + ceftazidime + gentamicin	Consider Candida
Acute pericarditis	S. pneumoniae, Staph aureus, gram-negative enteric rods	Cefotaxime or Ceftriaxone or Ceftizoxime	Enterovirus or "idiopathic" most common, consider M. tuberculosis
CENTRAL NERVOUS SYSTEM INFECTIONS			
Acute meningitis Age: 3 mos to 18 yrs	H. influenzae, S. pneumoniae, N. meningitidis	Cefotaxime/ceftriaxone/ceftizoxime	Culture, Gram stain, tests for antigen (pneumococcal, H. influenzae, meningococcal) may be helpful
Age: 18 yrs to 50 yrs	S. pneumoniae, N. meningitidis, H. influenzae	Cefotaxime/ceftriaxone/ceftizoxime or Ampicillin/penicillin	Also consider Lyme disease, acute HIV disease, syphilis, tuberculosis, fungal meningitis, Listeria
Age: over 50 yrs	S. pneumoniae, H. influenzae, N. meningitidis, Listeria monocytogenes, enteric gram-negative rods	Cefotaxime/ceftriaxone/ceftizoxime + ampicillin	As above

Post-trauma or postoperative	*S. pneumoniae, H. influenzae,* staphylococci (aureus and epidermidis), enteric gram-negative rods, (including pseudomonas)	Vancomycin + ceftazidime	
Shunt-associated	Staphylococci (coagulase-negative and aureus), *Propionibacterium acnes,* gram-negative enteric rods and enterococci	Vancomycin + ceftazidime ± rifampin	Shunt often must be removed
Encephalitis	*Herpes simplex* (most common of identified viruses)	Acyclovir	A long list of viral, rickettsial, and bacterial pathogens may cause encephalitis See AIDS infections for etiologies in AIDS patients
Brain abscess	Streptococci (*S. milleri* group), Bacteroides sp., enteric gram-negative rods, *Staph aureus*	Cefotaxime/ceftriaxone/ceftizoxime + metronidazole or Ceftazidime + metronidazole + vancomycin	Use ceftazidime regimen if pseudomonas suspected
Subdural empyema	As above plus *H. influenzae*	As above	
Epidural abscess	As above, staphylococci frequent	As above	
Suppurative intracranial phlebitis	As above, staphylococci frequent	As above	

SKIN AND SOFT TISSUE INFECTION

Impetigo	*S. pyogenes* and/or *Staph aureus*	Penicillin or Cloxacillin/dicloxacillin or Cephalexin/cefadroxil/cephradine or Erythromycin or Topical mupirocin	

(Continues)

Syndrome	Likely Disease or Pathogen	Therapy	Comment
Bullous impetigo	*Staph aureus*	Cloxacillin/dicloxacillin or Cephalexin	
Folliculitis	*Staph aureus*	Cloxacillin/dicloxacillin or Cephalexin/cefadroxil/cephradine	Consider pseudomonas with hot tub and pool exposure
Furuncles and carbuncles	*Staph aureus*	As above	
Erysipelas	*S. pyogenes*	Penicillin or Cephalexin/cefadroxil/cephradine or Cefazolin or Erythromycin	Rarely *Staph aureus*
Cellulitis	*S. pyogenes* or *Staph aureus*	Nafcillin/oxacillin/cloxacillin/dicloxacillin or Cephalexin/cefadroxil/cephradine or Cefazolin or Erythromycin	
Cellulitis with seafood or salt water exposure	*Vibrio sp.*	Piperacillin/mezlocillin/azlocillin/ticarcillin All + doxycycline/tetracycline/chloramphenicol	
Cellulitis with fresh water exposure	*Aeromonas sp.*	Trimethoprim-sulfamethoxazole or Ciprofloxacin Both ± gentamicin	
Diabetic foot infection	Usually mixed, with *Staph aureus*, *Staph epidermidis*, streptococci,	Cefoxitin/cefotetan/cefmetazole All ± gentamicin	Consider evaluation for bone involvement

	gram-negative rods, anaerobes	or Imipenem or Ceftazidime + metronidazole or Ciprofloxacin/ofloxacin + metronidazole or Ticarcillin-clavulanate ± gentamicin	
Infectious gangrene	Streptococci, anaerobic cocci, clostridia	Penicillin ± metronidazole	Debridement essential
Anaerobic cellulitis, necrotizing cellulitis, necrotizing fasciitis	Clostridial sp., other anaerobes gram-negative enteric rods	Penicillin + metronidazole + cefotaxime/ceftriaxone/ ceftizoxime/cefoperazone/ ceftazidime or Imipenem	gram-negatives seen in diabetics, debridement essential
Pyomyositis	Staph aureus	Nafcillin/oxacillin or Vancomycin or Cefazolin	Other organisms rarely may cause syndrome
Gas gangrene	C. perfringens, gram-negative enteric rods in some cases	Penicillin + cefotaxime/ceftriaxone/ ceftizoxime/ceftazidime/ cefoperazone or Imipenem or Chloramphenicol	Debridement needed, Gram stain helpful
Acute regional lymphadenitis	S. pyogenes, Staph aureus	Oxacillin/cloxacillin/natcillin or Cephalexin/cephradine/cefadroxil or Erythromycin	Also consider mycobacteria, cat scratch disease, lymphogranuloma venereum, chancroid

(Continues)

Syndrome	Likely Disease or Pathogen	Therapy	Comment
Lymphangitis, acute	*Strep pyogenes*	Penicillin or Erythromycin	Consider *S. aureus, Pasteurella multocida* (filariasis in tropical regions)
Lymphangitis, chronic	*Sporothrix schenckii, Mycobacterium marinum*	Potassium iodide for sporotrichosis rifampin + ethambutol for *M. marinum*	Biopsy and culture usually required
TRAUMA-RELATED INFECTIONS			
Burn sepsis	*Staph aureus, Enterobacter sp., S. pyogenes, Enterococcus faecalis, E. coli, P. aeruginosa*	Ceftazadime + vancomycin or Ticarcillin/piperacillin/mezlocillin/ azlocillin or aztreonam All + vancomycin + gentamicin/amikacin	Methicillin resistant staph may be a problem, infecting organisms different in different localities, therapy by clysis used in some centers, gram-positive also treated with topical silver sulfadiazine and gram-negative infections with mafenide acetate (Sulfamylon), consider *Candida albicans*
Dog/cat bite	*Pasteurella multocida, Staphylococci* (coagulase-negative and coagulase-positive), streptococci, *Bacteroides sp., Fusobacteria sp.*	Amoxicillin-clavulanate or Ampicillin-sulbactam or Tetracycline	Consider DF-2 (*Capnocytophaga canimorsus*) from dogs—may be lethal in splenectomized patients, consider tetanus prophylaxis
Human bite	Streptococci, *S. aureus, H. parainfluenzae, K. pneumoniae, Eikenella corrodens, Bacteroides sp., Fusobacterium sp.,* anaerobic cocci	Amoxicillin-clavulanate or Penicillin + cloxacillin/ dicloxacillin/oxacillin or Ampicillin-sulbactam	Consider tetanus prophylaxis
GASTROINTESTINAL INFECTIONS			
Acute inflammatory diarrhea	*Campylobacter jejuni, Shigella sp.,*	Ciprofloxacin/ofloxacin/norfloxacin	consider *C. difficile* (antibiotic-

(often with fever and fecal leukocytes)	*Salmonella sp.*, invasive *E. coli*	or Trimethoprim-sulfamethoxazole ± erythromycin	associated colitis) and amebic colitis, fluid replacement essential
Acute noninflammatory diarrhea	Toxigenic *E. coli*, rotavirus, norwalk-like viruses	Either no treatment or Ciprofloxacin/ofloxacin/norfloxacin or Trimethoprim-sulfamethoxazole	
Diarrhea of travelers	Toxigenic *E. coli*, and less often other pathogens listed above	Ciprofloxacin/norfloxacin/ofloxacin or Trimethoprim-sulfamethoxazole	Consider amebic colitis, loperamide may be helpful
Antibiotic associated colitis (pseudomembranous colitis)	*Clostridium difficile*	Oral metronidazole or Oral vancomycin	If possible, discontinue other antibiotics, avoid motility decreasing agents
Tropical sprue	Unknown	Tetracycline	Also PO folic acid and IM vitamin B_{12}

BONE AND JOINT INFECTIONS

Acute arthritis (children)	*Staph aureus, H. influenzae*, streptococci, gram-negative bacilli	Cefotaxime/ceftriaxone/ceftizoxime	Consider Lyme disease
Acute arthritis (adults)	*Staph aureus, N. gonorrhoeae*, gram-negative bacilli	Ceftriaxone/cefotaxime/ceftizoxime or Imipenem	Consider Lyme disease
Prosthetic joint infection	*Staph aureus, Staph epidermidis*, streptococci, gram-negative rods	Await identification of infecting organism or Vancomycin + ceftazidime	Joint usually must be removed, Gram stain and culture essential
Osteomyelitis, acute hematogenous	*Staph aureus*, also consider gram-negative rods	Nafcillin/oxacillin or Cefotaxime/ceftriaxone/ceftizoxime	Consider salmonella with sickle cell disease

(Continues)

Syndrome	Likely Disease or Pathogen	Therapy	Comment
Osteomyelitis with contiguous infection	*Staph aureus*, may be mixed with gram-negative rods and anaerobes	Nafcillin/oxacillin + gentamicin or Cefotaxime/ceftriaxone/ceftizoxime or Ciprofloxacin/ofloxacin All + metronidazole	Consider bone biopsy
Osteomyelitis with vascular insufficiency	Usually mixed, with *Staph aureus*, *Staph epidermidis*, streptococci, gram-negative rods, anaerobes	Cefoxitin/cefotetan/ cefmetazole all ± gentamicin or Imipenem or Ciprofloxacin/ofloxacin + metronidazole or Ticarcillin-clavulanate ± gentamicin	Consider bone biopsy
SEXUALLY TRANSMITTED DISEASES			
Urethritis	*N. gonorrhoeae, C. trachomatis*	Ceftriaxone (250 mg IM once) + doxycycline (100 mg PO bid x 7 days) or Ciprofloxacin (500 mg PO once)/ ofloxacin(400 mg PO once) + doxycycline (100 mg PO bid x 7 days) or Ofloxacin (300 mg PO bid x 7 days)	Consider syphilis and HIV infection
Epididymitis	*N. gonorrhoeae, C. trachomatis*	Ceftriaxone (250 mg IM once) + doxycycline (100 mg PO bid x 10 days)	
Cervicitis	*N. gonorrhoeae, C. trachomatis*	As above for urethritis	Consider syphilis and HIV infection
Pelvic Inflammatory disease	*N. gonorrhoeae, C. trachomatis*, gram-negative rods, anaerobes	Cefoxitin/cefotetan All + doxycycline or Clindamycin + gentamicin	Remove IUD

Prostatitis	See urinary tract infection		
Bacterial vaginosis	Alteration of flora, associated with *Gardnerella vaginalis* and *Mobiluncus sp.*	Metronidazole 500 mg PO (bid x 7 days)	Positive amine odor test, pH > 4.5, clue cells

EYE INFECTIONS

Conjunctivitis (children)	*H. influenzae, S. pneumoniae, Staph aureus,* adenovirus	Usually self-limited, topical gentamicin (gram-negative infections) or Topical neomycin/polymyxin	Consider trachoma in certain native American populations, Gram stain helpful
Conjunctivitis (adults)	*S. pneumoniae, Staph aureus,* adenovirus	As above	
Keratitis	*Staph aureus, S. pneumoniae, P. aeruginosa, Herpes simplex, Herpes zoster*	Specific therapy essential, often including topical, subconjunctival and parenteral administration	Obtain ophthalmologic consultation
Endophthalmitis	A long list of bacteria, fungi, viruses and parasites, *Staph aureus* and *P. aeruginosa,* most common following trauma or surgery	Attempt specific diagnosis, systemic and intravitreal gentamicin/amikacin AII + cefotaxime/ceftizoxime	Ophthalmologic consultation essential
Blepharitis/hordeola (sties)	*Staph aureus, Staph epidermidis*	Topical bacitracin or Sulfacetamide/erythromycin	Warm compresses
Orbital cellulitis	*Staph aureus, S. pneumoniae, S. pyogenes*	Natcillin/oxacillin or Cefotaxime/ceftriaxone/ceftizoxime	Beware of cavernous sinus infection and thrombosis, *H. influenzae* seen in children, CT scan helpful

Section 3

PREFERRED THERAPY FOR SPECIFIC PATHOGENS

BACTERIA, CHLAMYDIA, RICKETTSIA, AND RELATED ORGANISMS

Organism	Syndrome	Preferred Drugs	Also Effective
Acinetobacter calcoaceticus	Serious infection	Imipenem	Ticarcillin/ mezlocillin/ azlocillin *or* Ceftazidime All + gentamicin
	Urinary tract infection	Ciprofloxacin/ norfloxacin	Trimethoprim- sulfamethoxazole
Actinomyces israelii, naeslundii, viscosus, odontolyticus	Actinomycosis	Penicillin G	Tetracycline
Aeromonas species	Diarrhea, sepsis, cutaneous infection	Trimethoprim- sulfamethoxazole	Ciprofloxacin *or* Imipenem
Anthrax (see Bacillus anthracis)			
Arachnia propionica	Actinomycosis	Penicillin G	Tetracycline
Bacillus anthracis	Anthrax	Penicillin G	Erythromycin *or* Tetracycline
Bacillus cereus, subtilis	Serious infection	Vancomycin	Imipenem
Bacteroides fragilis	Intra-abdominal sepsis	Metronidazole *or* Imipenem	Clindamycin *or* Ticarcillin- clavulanate *or* Ampicillin-sulbactam *or* Cefoxitin/ cefmetazole/ cefotetan

Organism	Syndrome	Preferred Drugs	Also Effective
fragilis group distasonis, ovatus, thetaiotamicron	Intra-abdominal sepsis	Metronidazole *or* Imipenem	Chloramphenicol *or* Ticarcillin-clavulanate *or* Ampicillin-sulbactam
melaninogenicus	Lung abscess, orofacial infections	Clindamycin *or* Metronidazole	Imipenem *or* Cefoxitin/ cefotetan/ cefmetazole *or* Ampicillin/ penicillin G
Bordetella pertussis	Whooping cough	Erythromycin	Trimethoprim-sulfamethoxazole
Borrelia burgdorferi	Lyme borreliosis Early disease	Tetracycline/ doxycycline	Penicillin G/ amoxicillin *or* Erythromycin
	Late disease	Ceftriaxone/ cefotaxime	Penicillin G
recurrentis	Relapsing fever	Doxycycline/ tetracycline	Erythromycin
Branhamella (see Moraxella)			
Brucella species	Brucellosis	Doxycycline + rifampin	Doxycycline/ tetracycline + streptomycin *or* Trimethoprim-sulfamethoxazole + rifampin

(Continues)

Organism	Syndrome	Preferred Drugs	Also Effective
Calymmatobacterium granulomatis	Granuloma inguinale	Tetracycline/doxycycline	Trimethoprim-sulfamethoxazole *or* Chloramphenicol *or* Gentamicin
Campylobacter fetus	Serious infection	Imipenem	Gentamicin
jejuni	Diarrhea	Ciprofloxacin/norfloxacin/ofloxacin	Erythromycin *or* Tetracycline
Capnocytophaga canimorsus (DF2)	Periodontal sepsis, dog bite	Penicillin G	Erythromycin *or* Cefazolin *or* Clindamycin
Chlamydia pneumoniae (TWAR agent)	Pneumonia	Tetracycline	Erythromycin *or* Ofloxacin
psittaci	Psittacosis	Tetracycline	Chloramphenicol
trachomatis	Lymphogranuloma venerum	Doxycycline	Tetracycline *or* Erythromycin *or* Sulfisoxazole
	Trachoma	Oral and topical tetracycline	Oral and topical sulfa
	Urethritis, cervicitis, epididymitis	Tetracycline/doxycycline/minocycline	Erythromycin *or* Ofloxacin
Citrobacter diversus, freundii	Urinary tract infection	Ciprofloxacin/norfloxacin/ofloxacin	Gentamicin
	Pneumonia, serious infection	Imipenem	Aztreonam ± gentamicin

Organism	Syndrome	Preferred Drugs	Also Effective
Clostridium difficile	Diarrhea	Oral vancomycin *or* Oral metronidazole	Oral bacitracin
species	Gas gangrene, serious infection	Penicillin G	Metronidazole *or* Clindamycin *or* Imipenem *or* Tetracycline *or* Chloramphenicol
Corynebacterium Jeikeium (JK)	Serious infection	Vancomycin	
diphtheriae	Diphtheria	Erythromycin + antitoxin	Penicillin G + antitoxin
Coxiella burnetii	Q fever	Doxycycline/ tetracycline	Ciprofloxacin
DF2 (see Capnocyto- phaga canimorsus)			
Ehrlichia	Ehrlichiosis	Tetracycline/ doxycycline	
Eikenella corrodens	Oral infections	Ampicillin/ penicillin	Tetracycline *or* Erythromycin
Enterobacter	Serious infection	Gentamicin + ceftriaxone/ cefotaxime/ ceftizoxime/ *or* Imipenem	Piperacillin/ ticarcillin/ mezlocillin/ azlocillin/ Aztreonam *or* Ciprofloxacin All ± gentamicin
	Urinary tract infection	Trimethoprim- sulfamethoxazole *or* Ciprofloxacin/ norfloxacin/ ofloxacin	Nitrofurantoin *or* Tetracycline

(Continues)

Organism	Syndrome	Preferred Drugs	Also Effective
Enterococcus faecalis	Urinary tract infection	Ampicillin	Nitrofurantoin or Ciprofloxacin/ norfloxacin/ ofloxacin
	Endocarditis (check for high level gentamicin resistance)	Ampicillin + gentamicin	Vancomycin + gentamicin
Erysipelothrix rhusiopathiae	Cellulitis	Ampicillin	Tetracycline
	Endocarditis	Ampicillin + gentamicin	
Escherichia coli	Urinary tract infection	Trimethoprim-sulfamethoxazole or Ciprofloxacin/ norfloxacin/ ofloxacin	Nitrofurantoin or Trimethoprim
	Serious infection	Ceftriaxone/ cefotaxime/ ceftizoxime/ ceftazidime All ± gentamicin	Imipenem or Aztreonam or Ciprofloxacin
Flavobacterium meningosepticum	Sepsis	Vancomycin	Trimethoprim-sulfamethoxazole
Francisella tularensis	Tularemia	Gentamicin	Tetracycline
Fusobacterium species	Oral infection	Penicillin G	Cefoxitin or Imipenem or Metronidazole or Clindamycin

Organism	Syndrome	Preferred Drugs	Also Effective
Gonorrhea (see Neisseria gonorrhoeae)			
Haemophilus aphrophilus	Endocarditis	Ampicillin + gentamicin	
ducreyi	Chancroid	Ceftriaxone *or* Erythromycin	Trimethoprim-sulfamethoxazole *or* Amoxicillin-clavulanate *or* Ciprofloxacin
influenzae	Serious infection pneumonia, cellulitis	Ceftriaxone/ ceftizoxime/ cefotaxime *or* Chloramphenicol	Ampicillin (if β-lactamase negative) *or* Cefuroxime
	Meningitis	Ceftriaxone/ cefotaxime *or* Chloramphenicol	Ampicillin (if β-lactamase negative)
	Otitis, sinusitis	Amoxicillin-clavulanate *or* Cefuroxime *or* Cefuroxime axetil *or* Ceftriaxone/ ceftizoxime/ cefotaxime	Trimethoprim-sulfmethoxazole *or* Cefaclor/ cefadroxil/ cephradine *or* Cefixime

(Continues)

Organism	Syndrome	Preferred Drugs	Also Effective
Klebsiella pneumoniae	Urinary tract infection	Trimethoprim-sulfamethoxazole *or* Ciprofloxacin/ norfloxacin/ ofloxacin	Nitrofurantoin *or* Tetracycline
	Pneumonia	Ceftriaxone/ cefotaxime/ ceftizoxime/ ceftazidime ± gentamicin	Cefazolin/ *or* Imipenem *or* Ticarcillin-clavulanate *or* Aztreonam *or* Ampicillin-sulbactam *or* Ciprofloxacin All ± gentamicin
Legionella	Legionnaire's disease	Erythromycin ± rifampin	Ciprofloxacin? (no established alternative)
Leptospira	Leptospirosis	Penicillin G	Tetracycline/ doxycycline
Listeria monocytogenes	Listeriosis	Ampicillin ± gentamicin	Trimethoprim-sulfamethoxazole
Lyme disease (see Borrelia burgdorferi)			
Moraxella catarrhalis (Branhamella catarrhalis)	Sinusitis, otitis, bronchitis	Trimethoprim-sulfamethoxazole *or* Amoxacillin-clavulanate *or* Cefuroxime *or* Cefuroxime axetil	Tetracycline *or* Erythromycin/ clarithromycin *or* Cefaclor *or* Cefixime

Organism	Syndrome	Preferred Drugs	Also Effective
other species	Serious infection	Ampicillin/ penicillin G ± gentamicin	For β-lactamase positive strains use ceftriaxone/ cefotaxime/ ceftizoxime
Mycobacterium tuberculosis	Tuberculosis	Isoniazid + rifampin ± 2 months of pyrazinamide	Combinations including streptomycin, ethambutol, capreomycin, ethionamide
kansasii	Pneumonia	Isoniazid + rifampin ± ethambutol	Combinations including streptomycin, ethionamide, cycloserine, amikacin
leprae	Leprosy	Dapsone + rifampin ± clofazimine	Combinations including ethionamide *or* prothionamide
marinum	Subcutaneous infection	Rifampin + ethambutol	Minocycline
Mycoplasma pneumoniae	Pneumonia	Erythromycin	Tetracycline *or* Clarithromycin
Neisseria gonorrhoeae (gonococcus)	Urethritis, cervicitis, salpingitis	Ceftriaxone	Spectinomycin *or* Ciprofloxacin *or* Ofloxacin
	Disseminated	Ceftriaxone/ ceftizoxime/ cefotaxime	Spectinomycin

(Continues)

Organism	Syndrome	Preferred Drugs	Also Effective
meningitidis (meningococcus)	Meningitis	Penicillin G/ ampicillin (susceptible strains)	Chloramphenicol *or* Ceftriaxone/ cefotaxime
Nocardia	Pneumonia	Trimethoprim- sulfamethoxazole *or* Sulfisoxazole	Minocycline
Pasteurella multocida	Cat bite, arthritis, sepsis	Penicillin G/ ampicillin	Tetracycline *or* Ceftriaxone/ cefoperazone *or* Chloramphenicol
Pasteurella pestis (see Yersinia)			
Peptostreptococcus	Abscess	Penicillin G	Vancomycin *or* Clindamycin
Plague (see Yersinia pestis)			
Proteus mirabilis	Urinary tract infection	Ampicillin	Trimethoprim- sulfamethoxazole *or* Ciprofloxacin/ norfloxacin/ ofloxacin *or* Nitrofurantoin

Organism	Syndrome	Preferred Drugs	Also Effective
other species	Urinary tract	Ciprofloxacin/ norfloxacin/ ofloxacin	Trimethoprim-sulfamethoxazole *or* Nitrofurantoin
	Serious infection	Ceftriaxone/ cefotaxime/ ceftizoxime/ ceftazidime ± gentamicin	Ticarcillin/ azlocillin/ piperacillin/ mezlocillin *or* Aztreonam *or* Imipenem All ± gentamicin
Providencia stuarti	Serious infection	Ceftriaxone/ cefotaxime/ ceftizoxime ± gentamicin	Imipenem *or* Trimethoprim-sulfamethoxazole
	Urinary tract infection	Ciprofloxacin/ norfloxacin/ ofloxacin	Trimethoprim-sulfamethoxazole
Pseudomonas aeruginosa	Urinary tract infection	Ciprofloxacin/ norfloxacin/ ofloxacin	Indanyl carbenicillin
	Serious infection	Ticarcillin/ mezlocillin/ azlocillin/ piperacillin All + gentamicin	Ceftazidime/ cefoperazone *or* Aztreonam *or* Imipenem *or* Ciprofloxacin All + gentamicin
cepacia	Serious infection	Trimethoprim-sulfamethoxazole	Ceftazidime *or* Chloramphenicol

(Continues)

Organism	Syndrome	Preferred Drugs	Also Effective
maltophilia (see Xanthomonas)			
pseudomallei	Melioidosis	Ceftazidime	Combinations including Trimethoprim-sulfamethoxazole *or* Imipenem *or* Doxycycline *or* Chloramphenicol
Q fever (see Coxiella burnetii)			
Rhodococcus equi	Lung abscess	Vancomycin	Combinations including erythromycin *or* Gentamicin *or* Chloramphenicol *or* Trimethoprim-sulfamethoxazole
Rickettsia	Spotted fever, murine or endemic typhus, rickettsialpox	Doxycycline/ tetracycline	Chloramphenicol
Salmonella typhi	Typhoid fever	Trimethoprim-sulfamethoxazole *or* Ceftriaxone	Ciprofloxacin/ ofloxacin *or* Chloramphenicol *or* Amoxicillin/ ampicillin

Organism	Syndrome	Preferred Drugs	Also Effective
Serratia marcescens	Serious infection	Ceftriaxone/ ceftizoxime/ cefotaxime/ ceftazidime *or* Ciprofloxacin ± gentamicin	Aztreonam *or* Impenem *or* Piperacillin/ticarcillin/ azlocillin/ mezlocillin All ± gentamicin
	Urinary tract infection	Ciprofloxacin/ norfloxacin/ ofloxacin	Trimethoprim-sulfamethoxazole
Shigella	Dysentery	Ciprofloxacin/ norfloxacin	Trimethoprim-sulfamethoxazole (non-USA often resistant)
Spirillum minus	Rat bite fever (Sodoku)	Penicillin G	Doxycycline
Staphylococcus aureus methicillin-susceptible	Skin infection	Dicloxacillin/ cloxacillin	Cephalexin/ cephadroxil/ cephradine *or* Amoxicillin-clavulanate
	Serious infection	Oxacillin/ nafcillin/ *or* Vancomycin	Cefazolin/ cephalothin *or* Imipenem *or* Clindamycin
methicillin-resistant		Vancomycin	Teicoplanin *or* Ciprofloxacin + rifampin *or* Fusidic acid
Staphylococcus epidermidis	Serious infection	Vancomycin	Teicoplanin
Streptobaccillus moniliformis	Rat bite fever (Haverhill fever)	Penicillin G	Doxycycline *or* Streptomycin

(Continues)

Organism	Syndrome	Preferred Drugs	Also Effective
Streptococcus			
agalactiae (group B)	Serious infection	Penicillin G/ ampicillin ± gentamicin	Vancomycin *or* Ceftriaxone/ cefotaxime/ ceftizoxime All ± gentamicin
pneumoniae (pneumococcus)	Serious infection, pneumonia	Penicillin G *or* For penicillin-resistant, vancomycin	Cefuroxime/ cefazolin/ cephapirin *or* Erythromycin *or* Clindamycin
	Meningitis	Penicillin G	Ceftriaxone/ cefotaxime *or* Chloramphenicol
pyogenes (group A)	Pharyngitis	Penicillin V	Erythromycin/ clarithromycin
	Serious infection	Penicillin G	Cefazolin/ cephradine/ cefuroxime *or* Vancomycin *or* Clindamycin
viridans group or bovis	Endocarditis	Penicillin + streptomycin/ gentamicin	Vancomycin *or* Cefazolin All ± streptomycin/ gentamicin
Syphilis (see Treponema pallidum)			
Treponema pallidum	Early or late syphilis	Benzathine penicillin	Doxycycline *or* Tetracycline
	Neurosyphilis	IV penicillin G	Procaine penicillin + probenicid

Organism	Syndrome	Preferred Drugs	Also Effective
Tularemia (see Francisella tularensis)			
Ureaplasma urealyticum	Urethritis, cervicitis	Erythromycin	Doxycycline
Vibrio cholerae	Cholera	Tetracycline	Trimethoprim-sulfamethoxazole *or* Ciprofloxacin
Vibrio vulnificus	Serious infection	Tetracycline	Chloramphenicol *or* Penicillin G
Whipples' disease		Penicillin + streptomycin	Trimethoprim-sulfamethoxazole *or* Tetracycline
Whooping cough (see Bordetella pertusis)			
Xanthomonas maltophilia	Serious infection	Trimethoprim-sulfamethoxazole	Ticarcillin-clavulanate
Yersinia enterocolitica	Serious infection	Cefotaxime/ ceftizoxime/ ceftazidime *or* Gentamicin	Trimethoprim-sulfamethoxazole *or* Doxycycline *or* Chloramphenicol
pestis	Plague	Streptomycin	Tetracycline
	Plague meningitis	Chloramphenicol	

See Section 8 for dosages.
Caution: susceptibility of some organisms varies considerably between institutions.
Aminoglycosides: gentamicin is listed whenever an aminoglycoside is indicated because this drug is presently the least expensive and the most readily assayed for blood concentrations. Tobramycin or amikacin should be used instead when local susceptibility or price favors one of these.
Cephalosporins: only representative compounds are listed.

FUNGI (SEE AIDS SECTION FOR HIV-ASSOCIATED MYCOSES)

Deep Mycoses

Fungus	Drug
Aspergillus, invasive	Amphotericin B
Blastomyces dermatitidis rapidly progressing or meningeal	Amphotericin B
indolent, nonmeningeal	Ketoconazole/itraconazole[a]
Candida species	Amphotericin B ± flucytosine
Chromomycosis, agents of	Flucytosine
Coccidioides immitis, disseminated rapidly progressing	Amphotericin B
indolent	Ketoconazole/itraconazole[a]
meningeal	Intrathecal injection amphotericin B or miconazole *or* Oral fluconazole
Cryptococcus neoformans	Amphotericin B ± flucytosine
Histoplasma capsulatum	
chronic pulmonary or indolent, nonmeningeal disseminated infection	Ketoconazole/itraconazole[a]
disseminated infection in immunosuppressed patients	Amphotericin B
Mucormycosis, agents of	Amphotericin B
Pseudallescheria boydii	Ketoconazole/itraconazole[a]
Sporotrichosis lymphocutaneous	Oral iodides *or* Itraconazole[a]
extracutaneous	Amphotericin B

[a]Investigational in USA.

Superficial Mycoses

Vulvovaginal and Cutaneous Candidiasis

Drug	Vaginal Cream		Tablet/Suppository		Cutaneous Cream[b]
	Concentration (%)	Days	mg	Days	
Amphotericin B	–	–	–	–	+
Butoconazole	2	3 or 6[c]	–	–	–
Clotrimazole	1	7–14	100	7[d]	+
Clotrimazole	–	–	500	1	
Econazole	–	–	–	–	+
Ketoconazole	–	–	–	–	+
Miconazole	2	7	100	7	+
Miconazole	–	–	200	3	
Nystatin	–	–	100,000 U	14	+
Terconazole	0.4	7	80	3	–
Tioconazole	6.5	1	–	–	–

Columns: Vulvovaginitis[a] spans Vaginal Cream and Tablet/Suppository.

[a]All vaginal drugs are given as a single dose of cream or suppository inserted high in the vaginal vault upon retiring. Vaginal creams contain the recommended dose in 5 g.
[b]Some drugs are also available as lotions, powders, or solutions.
[c]Recommended duration for pregnant patients is 6 days.
[d]In nonpregnant women, two 100 mg tablets can be used each night for 3 days.

Oral Candidiasis

Drug	Dosage Form	Dose
Clotrimazole	10 mg troches	10 mg 5 times/day
Fluconazole	50 or 100 mg tabs	50-100 mg once daily
Ketoconazole	200 mg tabs	200-400 mg once daily
Nystatin	100,000 U/ml	5 ml 4 times/day

Treatment is usually continued for 14 days with all drugs.

Dermatophyes (Ringworm)

Systemic therapy
Griseofulvin (preferred systemic drug)
Microcrystalline
125 or 250 mg capsules
250 or 500 mg tablets: 500 to 1000 mg once daily
Ultramicrocrystalline
125, 250, or 330 mg capsules: 330 to 660 mg once daily
Ketoconazole
200 mg tablets: 200 to 400 mg once daily
Terbinafine
125, 250 mg capsules (not sold in USA): 250 mg bid
Topical formulations (creams, solutions, ointments, powders): ciclopirox
olamine, clotrimazole, econazole, haloprogin, ketoconazole, miconazole,
naftifine, undecylenate

PARASITES

Infection	Adult Regimen
Amoebiasis (Entamoeba histolytica) asymptomatic	Iodoquinol 650 mg PO tid for 20 days *or* Diloxanide furoate[a] 500 mg PO tid for 10 days *or* Paromomycin 500 mg PO tid for 7 days
dysentery, ameboma or liver abscess	Metronidazole 750 mg PO tid for 10 days followed by iodoquinol 650 mg tid for 20 days
Ascariasis (Ascaris lumbricoides)	Mebendazole 100 mg bid for 3 days *or* Pyrantel pamoate 11 mg/kg PO once (maximum 1 g)
Babesiosis (Babesia)	Clindamycin 600 mg IV or PO q8h together with quinine 650 mg PO tid for 7 days
Balantidiasis (Balantidium coli)	Tetracycline 500 mg PO qid for 10 days *or* Iodoquinol 650 mg PO tid for 20 days

Infection	Adult Regimen
Chaga's disease (see Trypanosomiasis)	
Clonorchis sinensis (see Flukes)	
Cryptosporidiosis	No proven effective therapy
Cysticercosis	Praziquantel 50 mg/kg/day divided into three doses, given for 14 days. In cerebral cysticercosis, short course corticosteroids are given to decrease cerebral reaction
Dientamoeba fragilis	Same as asymptomatic amoebiasis
Dracuncula medinensis	Metronidazole 250 mg PO tid for 10 days *or* Thiabendazole 50 mg/kg/day divided in 2 doses for 3 days
Echinococcosis (hydatid cyst)	No uniformly useful agent. Surgical resection of cyst may be useful. Also albendazole 400 mg PO bid for 28 days
Enterobiasis (pinworm)	Pyrantel pamoate 11 mg/kg PO once (maximum 1 g); repeat in 2 weeks *or* Mebendazole 100 mg PO once; repeat in 2 weeks
Fascioliasis (see Flukes)	
Filariasis (Wuchereria bancrofti, Brugia (W.) malayi, and Loa loa)	Diethylcarbamazine day 1: 50 mg PO once, day 2: 50 mg tid, day 3: 100 mg tid, days 4–21: 6 mg/kg/day in three divided doses after meals. Use 9 mg/kg/day in Loa loa
Onchocerca volvulus	Ivermectin[a] 150 µg/kg once. Repeat in 6–12 months
Flukes Clonorchis sinensis	Praziquantel 75 mg/kg/day PO in three divided doses for six doses
Fasciola hepatica	Bithionol[a] 30–50 mg/kg/day PO after meals in two or three divided doses on alternate days over 20–30 days
Fasciolopsis buski	Praziquantel 75 mg/kg/day PO in three divided doses for three doses
Opisthorchis viverrini	Praziquantel 75 mg/kg/day PO in three divided doses for three doses

(Continues)

Infection	Adult Regimen
Paragonimus westermani	Praziquantel 75 mg/kg/day PO in three divided doses for six doses
Giardiasis (Giardia lamblia)	Preferred: quinacrine 100 mg PO tid after meals for 5 days Alternate: metronidazole 250 mg PO tid for 7 days
Hookworm (Necator americanus or Ancylostoma duodenale)	Mebendazole 100 mg PO bid for 3 days *or* Pyrantel pamoate 11 mg/kg/day (maximum 1 g) for 3 days
Hydatid cyst (see Echinococcosis)	
Hymenolopis nana (see Tapeworm)	
Isosporiasis (Isospora belli)	Trimethoprim-sulfamethoxazole one double strength (160/800 mg) or two single strength (80/400 mg) qid for 10 days then bid for 3 weeks
Leishmaniasis: cutaneous, mucosal or visceral *(L. braziliensis, L mexicana, L donovani, L tropica, L major)*	Stibogluconate sodium[a] 20 mg antimony per kg in a single daily IV infusion. Treat cutaneous for 20 days and mucosal or visceral for 28 days. Courses may be repeated if necessary
Loa loa (see Filariasis)	

Malaria
  Chloroquine-resistant
  P falciparum
	Quinine sulfate 650 mg PO tid for 3 days (for cases acquired in Thailand give quinine for 7 days)
	or
	Quinidine gluconate 10 mg/kg loading (maximum 600 mg) in saline over 1 hour intravenously followed by continuous infusion of 0.02 mg/kg/min up to 3 days. Substitute oral quinine as soon as possible to complete 3 day course
	either of the above plus one of these
	Tetracycline 250 mg PO qid for 7 days
	or
	Pyrimethamine-sulfadoxine 3 tablets of 25/500 mg taken once on last day of quinine
	or
	Clindamycin 900 mg PO tid for 3 days
	For acute uncomplicated falciparum malaria, patients not already receiving quinine can be given: mefloquine 1250 mg once, with 8 oz water
	Caution: if quinine has been given, wait 12 hours before starting mefloquine

Infection	Adult Regimen
all other malaria	Chloroquine phosphate 1 g (600 mg chloroquine base) then 500 mg chloroquine phosphate 3 hours later, then another 500 mg at 24 and 48 hours. If intravenous therapy is required, use IV quinidine as stated above
prevention of relapse (P vivax and P ovale)	Primaquine phosphate 15 mg base (26.3 mg phosphate) daily for 14 days or 45 mg base once a week for 8 weeks. Screen for G6PD deficiency prior to use
prophylaxis	Mefloquine 250 mg PO once a week starting 1 week before travel and continuing 4 weeks after last exposure. Not recommended for Thailand *or* Doxycycline 100 mg daily *or* Chloroquine phosphate 500 mg (300 mg base) once a week beginning 1 week prior to travel and ending 4 weeks after last exposure, plus proguanil prophylaxis or pyrimethamine-sulfadoxine presumptive therapy as follows: proguanil (Paludrine) 200 mg daily during exposure and for 4 weeks afterwards. Widely available overseas. Useful in Africa south of the Sahara, or pyrimethamine-sulfadoxine (Fansidar): take 3 tablets (25/500 mg) once if otherwise unexplained febrile episode occurs. Fansidar is contraindicated in patients allergic to sulfonamides
Necator americanus (see Hookworm)	
Onchocerca (see Filariasis)	
Paragonimus (see Fluke)	
Pinworm (see Enterobius)	
Pneumocystis carinii	Trimethoprim-sulfamethoxazole 20/100 mg/kg/day IV or PO in three divided doses each day for 14–21 days. Maximum dose 2 DS tablets (320/1600 mg) q8h *or* Pentamidine isethionate 4 mg/kg IM or IV once a day for 14–21 days

(Continues)

Infection	Adult Regimen
Scabies	Drug of choice: 5% permethrin cream, spread over entire body; wash off after 8–14 hours *or* Lindane (Kwell) spread over body below neck, leave overnight then wash off Launder bedding and clothing at time of treatment
Schistosomiasis *S haematobium*	Praziquantel 40 mg/kg in two divided doses on 1 day
S japonicum	Praziquantel 60 mg/kg in three divided doses on 1 day
S mansoni	Preferred: praziquantel 40 mg/kg in two divided doses on 1 day *or* Oxamniquine 15 mg/kg PO once
S mekongi	Praziquantel 60 mg/kg in three divided doses on 1 day
Strongyloidiasis	Thiabendazole 50 mg/kg/day in two divided doses (maximum 3 g/day) on 2 days (treat hyperinfection syndrome for up to 2–3 weeks)
Tapeworm Diphyllobothrium latum, Dipyllidium caninum, Taenia saginata, Taenia solium	Niclosamide 2 g (4 tablets) chewed thoroughly and washed down with a little water, take after a light meal *or* Praziquantel 10–20 mg/kg once
Hymenolepis nana	Praziquantel 25 mg/kg once *or* Niclosamide 2 g daily for 6 days
Toxocariasis (see Visceral larva migrans)	
Toxoplasmosis	Pyrimethamine 25 mg once a day + sulfadiazine 4 g/day in four divided doses for 3–4 weeks

Infection	Adult Regimen
Trichinosis	Mebendazole 200–400 mg PO tid x 3d then 400–500 mg tid x 10d. Steroids are added for severe symptoms
Trichomoniasis	Metronidazole 40 mg/kg (maximum 2 g) PO once or 500 mg PO bid for 7 days
Trichostrongyliasis	Preferred: pyrantel pamoate 11 mg/kg once (maximum 1 g) Alternative: mebendazole 100 mg PO bid x 3d
Trichuriasis (whipworm)	Mebendazole 100 mg PO bid for 3 days
Trypanosomiasis	
T cruzi (Chagas' disease)	Nifurtimox[a] 8–10 mg/kg PO in four divided doses for 120 days

T brucei gambiensis,
  T brucei rhodesiense
  (Afican sleeping sickness)
	Early, hemolymphatic stage: suramin.[a] Start with 100–200 mg test dose IV. Then 20 mg/kg (maximum 1 g) IV (slow infusion) days 1, 3, 7, 14 and 21

	CNS stage: melarsoprol[a] 2-3.6 mg/kg/day IV in three divided doses for 3 days; wait 1 week then 3.6 mg/kg/day IV in three divided doses for 3 days; repeat course after 10–21 days. Toxic drug. See *PPID* for details
Visceral larva migrans	Diethylcarbamazine 6 mg/kg/day in three divided doses for 7–10 days *or* Thiabendazole 50 mg/kg/day in two divided doses for 5 days (maximum 3 g/day)
Whipworm (see Trichuriasis)	
Wuchereria bancrofti (see Filariasis)	

[a]Available in the USA from the Centers for Disease Control. Telephone 404-639-3670.
(Adapted from drugs for parasitic infections. Med Let 34:17, 1992, with permission.)

VIRUSES

ANTIVIRAL THERAPY

Virus	Infection	Drug of Choice	Alternative Drugs	Comments
Cytomegalovirus	Congenital	None proven		
	Gastroenteritis	None proven		
	Hepatitis	None proven		
	Pneumonia	Ganciclovir		Ganciclovir + hyperimmune globulin in bone marrow transplant recipients
	Retinitis	Ganciclovir	Foscarnet	AIDS patients: ganciclovir 5 mg/kg once daily as maintenance therapy useful
Hepatitis A virus	Acute hepatitis	None proven		
Hepatitis B virus	Chronic hepatitis	Interferon-α 2a or interferon-α 2b		
Hepatitis C virus	Chronic hepatitis	Interferon-α 2a or interferon-α 2b		
Herpes simplex virus type 1 or type 2	Encephalitis	Acyclovir IV	Vidarabine IV	High dose necessary for 10–14 days, acyclovir 10 mg/kg q8h IV, vidarabine 15 mg/kg q24h IV over 12 hours
	Genital, primary	Acyclovir oral		Treat only moderately severe cases; 200 mg PO 5 times/day x 10 days
	Genital, recurrent	Acyclovir oral		200 mg 5 times/day x 5 days
	Prophylaxis of frequent recurrence	Acyclovir oral		200 mg oral 2–5 times a day
	Keratoconjunctivitis topical	Trifluridine	Acyclovir topical or idoxuridine topical or vidarabine topical	
	Mucocutaneous, compromised host	Acyclovir oral or IV		
	Neonatal	Acyclovir IV		

Virus	Infection	Drug of Choice	Alternative Drugs	Comments
Human immunodeficiency virus		See page 90		
Influenza A virus	Influenza treatment	Amantadine	Rimantadine[a]	For 5–7 days
	Influenza virus pneumonia	None proven		
	Prophylaxis	Amantadine	Rimantadine[a]	For duration of exposure
Papillomavirus	Genital papilloma (condyloma acuminatum)	Interferon-α 2b intralesionally, intramuscularly, or subcutaneously		
Respiratory syncytial virus	Bronchiolitis ± pneumonia	Ribavirin aerosol		
Varicella zoster virus	Localized zoster			
	Immunocompromised host	Acyclovir IV[b]	Vidarabine IV	
	Normal host	Acyclovir IV *or* oral		Oral therapy requires high dose - 800 mg PO 5 times/day for 7–10 days
	Varicella (chicken pox)			
	Immunocompromised host	Acyclovir IV[b]	Vidarabine IV	
	Normal host	Acyclovir IV	Vidarabine IV	

[a]Investigational in USA.
[b]Adults 10 mg/kg IV q8h x 7 days; children 500 mg/m^2 IV q8h x 7 days
See section 8 for dosages.

Section 4

TREATMENT OF SEXUALLY TRANSMITTED DISEASES

Causative Organism and/or Type of Illness	Drug of Choice	Dosage	Alternatives
Chancroid	Erythromycin or Ceftriaxone	500 mg oral qid x 7 days 250 mg IM once	Trimethoprim-sulfamethoxazole 160/800 mg oral bid x 7 days or Ciprofloxacin 500 mg oral bid x 3 days
Chlamydia trachomatis			
Urethritis cervicitis, oculogenital syndrome and proctitis	Doxycycline	100 mg oral bid x 7 days	Ofloxacin 300 mg bid x 7 days or Erythromycin 500 mg oral qid x 7 days
Neonatal Ophthalmia	Erythromycin	12.5 mg/kg oral or IV qid x 14 days	Sulfisoxazole 100 mg/kg/day oral or IV in divided doses (after 4 weeks old) x 14 days
Pneumonia	Erythromycin	12.5 mg/kg oral or IV qid x 14 days	
Lymphogranuloma venereum	Doxycycline	100 mg oral bid x 21 days	Erythromycin 500 mg oral qid x 21 days
Epididymitis (sexually acquired)	Ceftriaxone followed by doxycycline	250 mg IM once 100 mg oral bid x 10 days	Ofloxacin 300 mg bid x 10 days (data limited)
Herpes simplex			
First episode genital	Acyclovir	200 mg oral 5 times/day x 7–10 days	Acyclovir 400 mg oral tid x 7–10 days
First episode proctitis	Acyclovir	400 mg oral 5 times/day x 7–10 days	Acyclovir 800 mg oral tid x 7–10 days
Severe	Acyclovir	5 mg/kg IV tid x 5–7 days	
Prevention of recurrences	Acyclovir	200 mg oral 2–5 times a day	Acyclovir 400 mg bid
Lymphogranuloma venerum	See under *Chlamydia trachomatis*		

Neisseria gonorrhoeae

Urethral, cervical, or rectal	Ceftriaxone	125–250 mg IM once	Spectinomycin 2 g IM once Ciprofloxacin 500 mg orally once Ofloxacin 400 mg orally once Cefixime 400 mg once PO
Pharyngeal	Ceftriaxone	125–250 mg IM once	Ciprofloxacin 500 mg orally once (limited data) Ofloxacin 400 mg orally once (limited data)
Ophthalmia (adults)	Ceftriaxone	1 g IM once plus saline irrigation	Ceftriaxone 1 g IV or IM daily x 5 days, plus saline irrigation
Disseminated gonococcal infection (DGI)	Ceftriaxone	1 g IV daily x 7–10 days	Ceftizoxime or cefotaxime, 1 g IV q8h for 2–3 days or until improved, followed by cefuroxime axetil 500 mg orally bid to complete 7–10 days total therapy
Neonatal Ophthalmia	Cefotaxime or Ceftriaxone	25 mg/kg IV or IM qh8–12h x 7 days, plus saline irrigation 125 mg IM once plus saline irrigation	Penicillin G 100,000 U/kg/day IV in 4 doses x 7 days plus saline irrigation (if susceptible)
Disseminated gonococcal infection	Cefotaxime	25–50 mg/kg IV q8–12h x 10–14 days	Penicillin G 100,000 U/kg/day IV in 4 doses x 7 days (if susceptible)
Meningitis	Cefotaxime	50 mg/kg IV q8–12h x 10–14 days	Penicillin G 150,000 U/kg/day IV in 4 doses for at least 10 days (if susceptible)
Children (under 45 kg) Urogenital, rectal, and pharyngeal	Ceftriaxone	125 mg IM once	Spectinomycin 40 mg/kg IM once (not for pharyngeal) Amoxicillin 50 mg/kg oral once plus probenecid 25 mg/kg (maximum 1 g) oral once (if susceptible, not for pharyngeal) Penicillin G procaine 100,000 U/kg IM once plus probenecid 25 mg/kg (maximum 1 g) oral once (if susceptible)

(Continues)

Causative Organism and/or Type of Illness	Drug of Choice	Dosage	Alternatives
Neisseria gonorrhoeae Children (under 45 kg)			
Arthritis	Ceftriaxone or Cefotaxime	50 mg/kg/day (max 2 g) IV x 7 days 50 mg/kg/day IV in divided doses x 7 days	Penicillin G 150,000 U/kg/day IV x 7 days (if susceptible)
Pelvic Inflammatory Disease			
Hospitalized patients	Cefoxitin or Cefotetan Either one plus Doxycycline followed by Doxycycline[a]	2 g IV q6h 2 g IV q12h 100 mg IV q12h until improved 100 mg oral bid to complete 10–14 days	Clindamycin 900 mg IV q8h plus gentamicin 2 mg/kg/IV once followed by gentamicin 1.5 mg/kg/IV q8h until improved followed by doxycycline[a] 100 mg oral bid to complete 10–14 days
Outpatients	Cefoxitin plus probenecid or Ceftriaxone Either one followed by Doxycycline[a]	2 g IM once 1 g oral once 250 mg IM once 100 mg oral bid x 10–14 days	
Syphilis			
Early (primary, secondary, or latent less than one year)	Penicillin G benzathine	2.4 million U IM once	Doxycycline[a] 100 mg oral bid x 2 weeks, Ceftriaxone 250 mg IM once daily x 10 days
Late (more than one year's duration, cardiovascular, gumma, late-latent)	Penicillin G benzathine	2.4 million U IM weekly x 3 weeks	Doxycycline[a] 100 mg oral bid x 4 weeks
Neurosyphilis	Penicillin G or Penicillin G procaine plus probenecid	2.4 million U IV q4h x 10–14 days 2.4 million U IM daily; 500 mg qid orally both x 14 days	No proven effective alternative
Congenital	Penicillin G or Penicillin G procaine	50,000 U/kg IV q8–12h for 10–14 days 50,000 U/kg IM daily for 10–14 days	

Vaginal Infection

Trichomoniasis	Metronidazole	2 g oral once or 500 mg oral bid x 7 days (avoid in pregnancy)	
Bacterial vaginosis	Metronidazole	500 mg oral bid x 7 days	Clindamycin 300 mg oral bid x 7 days
Vulvovaginal candidiasis	Miconazole nitrate	200 mg suppository intravaginally hs x 3 days	Miconazole nitrate (100 mg suppository or 5 g 2% cream) intravaginally hs x 7–14 days
	or Clotrimazole	100 mg vaginal tablets intravaginally two hs x 3 days	Clotrimazole (100 mg vaginal tablet or 5 g 1% cream) intravaginally hs x 7 days
	or Butoconazole	5 g of 2% cream intravaginally hs x 3 days	Butoconazole (5 g of 2% cream) intravaginally hs x 3–6 days
	or Terconazole	80 mg suppository intravaginally hs x 3 days	Terconazole (0.4% cream) 5 g intravaginally hs x 7 days

[a]Tetracycline 500 mg oral qid may be substituted for doxycycline 100 mg oral bid.
(Adapted from Treatment of Sexually Transmitted Diseases. Med Let 32:(810) 5–10, 1990, and CDC 1989 Sexually Transmitted Diseases Treatment Guidelines MMWR 38:(S–8)1, 1989, with permission.)
See section 2 for therapy of syndromes.

Section 5

THERAPY FOR HIV ASSOCIATED INFECTION

THERAPY OF PATIENTS INFECTED WITH THE HUMAN IMMUNODEFICIENCY VIRUS (HIV-1)

Antiretroviral Therapy

Patients with HIV-1 positive serology, a CD4 count below 500, and a prior episode of Pneumocystis pneumonia or other AIDS-defining opportunistic infection should receive zidovudine (AZT) 200 mg q4h (1200 mg/day) for 1 month followed by 100 mg 5 to 6 times per day.

For asymptomatic HIV infection and a CD4 count below 500 administer zidovudine 100 mg 5 times per day.

Patients intolerant of AZT may be given didanosine. See page 122 for dose.

Therapy for Opportunistic Infections

Candida albicans: Oropharyngeal or Esophageal

Clotrimazole 10 mg troche 5 times per day
   or
Ketoconazole 400 mg PO once daily. Not useful if patient is taking H_2 receptor blocking agent, omeprazine or rifampin
   or
Fluconazole 100 mg PO once daily
   or
Amphotericin B IV 0.25 mg/kg daily. Reserve for refractory, endoscopy-proven cases of esophagitis

Oropharyngeal candidiasis resolves in 7 to 10 days. Esophageal candidiasis is treated for at least 2 weeks after disappearance of symptoms. Recurrence in either site is usual

Cryptococcal Meningitis

Initial
   Amphotericin B 0.5 mg/kg IV once daily until cultures are negative and symptoms improve
      or

In patients with good prognosis, fluconazole 400 mg PO qd. Good prognostic signs include normal mentation, negative blood culture, serum antigen below 1:256, and negative India ink smear of cerebrospinal fluid (CSF)

Maintenance

Amphotericin B 1 mg/kg IV once a week

or

Fluconazole 200 mg PO once daily

Cytomegalovirus Retinitis: 2 Weeks Initial, then Maintenance

Ganciclovir 5 mg/kg IV q12h for 14–21 days then 5 mg/kg IV daily. Watch white blood cells (WBC), platelets

or

Foscarnet 60 mg/kg IV q8h for 21 days then 90 mg/kg daily. Watch renal function

Herpes Simplex

Mild mucocutaneous: acyclovir 200 to 400 mg PO 5 times/day

Severe mucocutaneous or esophageal infection: 5 mg/kg IV q8h for at least 7 days

Histoplasmosis, Disseminated

Initial

Amphotericin B 0.5 mg/kg IV daily for 6 weeks

Maintenance

Amphotericin B 1 mg/kg IV once a week

or

Itraconazole 200 mg PO once daily (investigational in USA)

Mycobacterium avium-intracellulare

No proven effective regimen. Consider amikacin 7.5 mg/kg daily for 4 weeks, plus ciprofloxacin 750 mg PO twice daily, plus ethambutol 15 mg/kg PO once daily (max 1 g) plus rifampin 10 mg/kg once daily (max 600 mg)

Mycobacterium Tuberculosis

Isoniazid 300 mg/day and rifampin 600 mg/day for 9 months with an initial 2 months that includes pyrazinamide 20 to 30 mg/kg daily (usual adult dose 2 g/day)

For meningitis or suspected drug resistance treat as above with ethambutol 25 mg/kg once daily for 6 weeks followed by 15 mg/kg once daily for 9 months

For PPD intermediate (5 tu) of at least 5 mm administer isoniazid 300 mg once daily for 12 months

Pneumocystis Pneumonia (PCP)

Initial 21 days

Trimethoprim-sulfamethoxazole 20/100 mg/kg IV or PO divided into 8-hour intervals. Maximum dose 2 DS (320/1600 mg) q8h. (Watch for severe rash, low WBC or platelets, and hepatitis.)

or

Pentamidine 4 mg/kg IV or IM once daily. (Watch for hypotension, azotemia, pancreatitis, hypoglycemia, diabetes mellitus, low WBC, fever, prolonged QT interval, and sterile abscess at IM injection sites.) Replace K and Mg as needed to minimize possibility of cardiac arrhythmia

or

For mild to moderately severe pneumonia: trimethoprim 20 mg/kg/day PO in three divided doses (max dose 300 mg PO tid) plus dapsone 100 mg PO once daily

or

For patients with PaO_2 <70 on room air or A-a gradient >30, consider adding prednisone 40 mg bid × 5 days, 40 mg qd × 5 days then 20 mg qd × 11 days. Untreated concomitant cryptococcosis, histoplasmosis, tuberculosis, or strongyloidiasis may be worsened by steroids

Maintenance after initial episode (PCP) or with CD4 count below 200

Trimethoprim 160 mg-sulfamethoxazole 800 mg (2 tabs or 1 DS) PO bid. One DS tablet three times a week may also be adequate

or

Pentamidine aerosol 300 mg once a month by Respirgard II nebulizer (Marquest, Englewood, CO)
> *or*

Dapsone 100 mg PO daily

Syphilis

Early syphilis
> Benzathine penicillin G 2.4 million units IM, three doses 1 week apart. Follow-up serum serologic testing at 1, 2, 3, 6, 9, and 12 months is important, with LP and retreatment indicated if titers fail to fall

Late or neurosyphilis
> Aqueous penicillin G 2 to 4 million units IV q4h for 10 days
> > *or*
>
> Procaine penicillin 2.4 million units IM once daily plus probenecid 500 mg PO 4 times a day for 10 to 14 days
>
> With all regimens, follow serologic tests for 3 years

Toxoplasmosis

Pyrimethamine is given as a loading dose of 200 mg followed by 50–100 mg PO qd + sulfadiazine 1–1.5 g PO q6h + folinic acid (not folate) 10 mg PO qd, continued indefinitely, with at least 2 L fluid intake daily to prevent sulfadiazine-induced crystalluria and oliguria. Sodium bicarbonate can be added to raise urine pH to at least 7.5, decreasing crytalluria. Watch WBC, platelets.

Sulfa allergic patients may be treated with clindamycin 1200 mg IV q6h or 600 mg PO q6–8h plus pyrimethamine 50–100 mg qd and folinic acid 10 mg PO qd for acute therapy or clindamycin 300 mg PO q6h or 450 mg PO q8h with pyrimethamine 25–50 mg PO qd for maintenance therapy.

Section 6

PROPHYLAXIS

PROPHYLAXIS FOR SURGICAL PROCEDURES

Surgical Procedure	Prophylactic Antimicrobials Indicated	Regimen
Biliary tract surgery		
High risk >70 years Obstructive jaundice Acute cholecystitis Cholangitis Common duct stone	yes	Cefazolin 1 g IV/IM once or Gentamicin 1.5 mg/kg IV preoperative and q8h x 3
Low risk	no	
Gynecologic surgery		
Hysterectomy Vaginal	yes	Cefazolin 1 g IV/IM then q8h x 2, or Cefoxitin 2 g IV then q4h x 2, or Cefotetan 2 g IV as single dose
Abdominal	yes	Cefazolin 1 g IV/IM then q8h x 2, or Cefoxitin 2 g IV then q4h x 2

Cesarean section		
High risk (premature rupture, etc.)	yes	Cefazolin 1 g IV/IM then q8h x 2, <u>or</u> Cefoxitin 2 g IV then q4h x 2, <u>or</u> Cefotetan 2 g IV as single dose
Low risk	no	
Therapeutic abortion		
Previous PID	yes	Aqueous penicillin G 1 million U preoperative <u>or</u>
Mid-trimester abortion	yes	Cefazolin 1 g IV/IM preoperative
Orthopaedics		
Open fracture	yes	Cefazolin 1 g q8h ± gentamicin 1.5 mg/kg IV q8h x 3 doses (alter per cultures)
Clean cases	no	
Prosthesis (joint replacement)	yes	Cefazolin 1 g IV/IM preoperative and q8h x 2 days <u>or</u> Vancomycin 1 g IV preoperative and 0.5 g q6h x 2 days
Amputation	yes	Cefoxitin 2 g IV preoperative and q6h for 4 doses

(Continues)

PROPHYLAXIS FOR SURGICAL PROCEDURES (*Continued*)

Surgical Procedure	Prophylactic Antimicrobials Indicated	Regimen
Gastrointestinal surgery		
Elective colorectal	yes	Oral (day before surgery): Neomycin 1 g plus erythromycin 1 g x 3 given at 1 p.m., 2 p.m., and 11 p.m.
Nonelective colorectal	yes	Parenteral: Cefoxitin 1 g IV and q8h x 3, <u>or</u> Cefotetan 2 g IV as single dose, <u>or</u> Clindamycin 600 mg IV plus gentamicin 1.5 mg/kg IV and q8h × 3, <u>or</u> Metronidazole 500 mg IV plus gentamicin 1.5 mg/kg IV and q8h x 3
Gastroduodenal surgery Bleeding or obstruction	yes	Cefazolin 1 g IV/IM preoperative
Appendectomy	yes	Cefoxitin 1-2 g IV preoperative and 1-5 days postoperative

Urologic surgery

Sterile urine — no

Positive urine culture — yes — Treat urinary tract infection with appropriate antibiotics

Head and neck operations

Uncontaminated — no

Incision through oral or pharyngeal mucous membranes — yes — Cefazolin 2 g IV/IM preoperative, <u>or</u> Clindamycin 600 mg IV plus gentamicin 1.5 mg/kg IV preoperative and q8h x 2

Thoracic surgery

Lobectomy, pneumonectomy — yes — Cefazolin 1 g IV and q8h x 2 days

Neurosurgery

CSF shunt — no

Craniotomy Routine — no

(Continues)

Surgical Procedure	Prophylactic Antimicrobials Indicated	Regimen
High-risk Re-exploration Microsurgery	yes	Vancomycin 1 g IV ± gentamicin 1.5 mg/kg IV
Cardiovascular surgery		
Open heart procedures Vascular	yes	Cefazolin or cefuroxime 1 g IV/IM then q8h x 1-2 days, or Vancomycin 1.0 g IV then 0.5 g q6h x 2 days
Coronary artery bypass grafting	yes	Cefazolin or cefuroxime 1 g IV/IM then q8h x 1-2 days, or Vancomycin 1.0 g IV then 0.5 g q6h x 2 days
Pacemaker insertion	no	Only in centers with high infection rate
Peripheral vascular surgery		
Reconstruction abdominal aorta	yes	Cefazolin or cefuroxime 1 g IV/IM then q8h x 1-2 days, or Vancomycin 1.0 g IV then 0.5 g q6h x 2 days
Vascular operation on leg with groin incision	yes	Cefazolin 1 g IV/IM then q8h x 1-2 days, or Vancomycin 1.0 g IV then 0.5 g q6h x 2 days

PROPHYLAXIS FOR BACTERIAL ENDOCARDITIS

Cardiac Conditions[a]

Endocarditis Prophylaxis Recommended

Prosthetic cardiac valves, including bioprosthetic and homograft valves
Previous bacterial endocarditis, even in the absence of heart disease
Most congenital cardiac malformations
Rheumatic and other acquired valvular dysfunction, even after valvular
 surgery
Hypertrophic cardiomyopathy
Mitral valve prolapse with valvular regurgitation

Endocarditis Prophylaxis Not Recommended

Isolated secundum atrial septal defect
Surgical repair without residua beyond 6 months of secundum atrial
 septal defect, ventricular septal defect, or patent ductus arteriosus
Previous coronary artery bypass graft surgery
Mitral valve prolapse without valvular regurgitation[b]
Physiologic, functional, or innocent heart murmurs
Previous Kawasaki disease without valvular dysfunction
Previous rheumatic fever without valvular dysfunction
Cardiac pacemakers and implanted defibrillators

[a]This table lists selected conditions but is not meant to be all-inclusive.
[b]Individuals who have a mitral valve prolapse associated with thickening
and/or redundancy of the valve leaflets may be at increased risk for
bacterial endocarditis, particularly men who are 45 years of age or
older.

(This section from Danjani AS, Bisno AL, Chung KJ et al: Prevention of bacterial endocarditis: Recommendations of the American Heart Association. JAMA 264:2919–2922,
1990, with permission.)

Dental or Surgical Procedures[a]

Endocarditis Prophylaxis Recommended

Dental procedures known to induce gingival or mucosal bleeding,
 including professional cleaning
Tonsillectomy and/or adenoidectomy
Surgical operations that involve intestinal or respiratory mucosa
Bronchoscopy with a rigid bronchoscope
Sclerotherapy of esophageal varices
Esophageal dilatation
Gallbladder surgery
Cytoscopy
Urethral dilatation
Urethral catheterization if urinary tract infection is present[b]
Urethral surgery if urinary tract infection is present[b]
Prostatic surgery
Incision and drainage of infected tissue[b]
Vaginal hysterectomy
Vaginal delivery in the presence of infection[b]

Endocarditis Prophylaxis Not Recommended[c]

Dental procedures not likely to induce gingival bleeding, such as simple
 adjustment of orthodontic appliances or fillings above the gum line
Injection of local intraoral anesthetic (except intraligamentary injections)
Shedding of primary teeth
Tympanostomy tube insertion
Endotracheal intubation
Bronchoscopy with a flexible bronchoscope, with or without biopsy
Cardiac catheterization
Endoscopy with or without gastrointestinal biopsy
Cesarean section
In the absence of infection; urethral catheterization, dilatation and
 curettage, uncomplicated vaginal delivery, therapeutic abortion,
 sterilization procedures, or insertion or removal of intrauterine devices

---

[a]This table lists selected conditions but is not meant to be all-inclusive.
[b]In addition to prophylactic regimen for genitourinary procedures, antibiotic therapy should
be directed against the most likely bacterial pathogen.
[c]In patients who have prosthetic heart valves, a previous history of endocarditis, or
surgically constructed systemic-pulmonary shunts or conduits, physicians may choose to
administer prophylactic antibiotics even for low-risk procedures that involve the lower
respiratory, genitourinary, or gastrointestinal tracts.

Recommended Prophylactic Regimen for Dental, Oral, or Upper Respiratory Tract Procedures in Patients Who Are at Risk[a]

Drug	Dosing Regimen[b]
Amoxicillin	3.0 g PO 1 h before procedure; then 1.5 g 6 h after initial dose
Amoxicillin/penicillin-allergic patients	
Erythromycin	Erythromycin ethylsuccinate, 800 mg, or erythromycin stearate, 1.0 g, PO 2 h before procedure; then half the dose 6 h after initial dose
Clindamycin	300 mg PO 1 h before procedure and 150 mg 6 h after initial dose

[a]Includes those with prosthetic heart valves and other high-risk patients.
[b]Initial pediatric doses are as follows: amoxicillin, 50 mg/kg; erythromycin ethylsuccinate or erythromycin stearate, 20 mg/kg; and clindamycin, 10 mg/kg. Follow-up doses should be one-half the initial dose. *Total pediatric dose should not exceed total adult dose.* The following weight ranges may also be used for the initial pediatric dose of amoxicillin: <15 kg, 750 mg; 15 to 30 kg, 1500 mg; and >30 kg, 3000 mg (full adult dose).

Alternate Prophylactic Regimens for Dental, Oral, or Upper Respiratory Tract Procedures in Patients Who Are at Risk

Drug	Dosing Regimen[a]
Patients unable to take oral medications	
Ampicillin	IV or IM administration of ampicillin, 2.0 g, 30 min before procedure; then IV or IM administration of ampicillin, 1.0 g, or oral administration of amoxicillin, 1.5 g, 6 h after initial dose
Ampicillin/amoxicillin/penicillin-allergic patients unable to take oral medication	
Clindamycin	IV administration of 300 mg 30 min before procedure and an IV or oral administration of 150 mg 6 h after initial dose
Patients considered high risk and not candidates for standard regimen	
Ampicillin, gentamicin, and amoxicillin	IV or IM administration of ampicillin, 2.0 g, plus gentamicin, 1.5 mg/kg (not to exceed 80 mg), 30 min before procedure; followed by amoxicillin, 1.5 g, PO 6 h after initial dose; alternatively, the parenteral regimen may be repeated 8 h after initial dose
Ampicillin/amoxicillin/penicillin-allergic patients considered high risk	
Vancomycin	IV administration of 1.0 g over 1 h, starting 1 h before procedure; no repeated dose necessary

[a]Initial pediatric doses are as follows: ampicillin, 50 mg/kg; clindamycin, 10 mg/kg; gentamicin, 2.0 mg/kg; vancomycin, 20 mg/kg. Follow-up doses should be one-half the initial dose. Total pediatric dose should not exceed total adult dose. No initial dose is recommended in this table for amoxicillin (25 mg/kg is the follow-up dose).

Regimens for Genitourinary/Gastrointestinal Procedures

Drug	Dosing Regimen[a]
Standard regimen	
Ampicillin, gentamicin, and amoxicillin	IV or IM administration of ampicillin, 2.0 g, plus gentamicin, 1.5 mg/kg (not to exceed 80 mg), 30 min before procedure; followed by amoxicillin, 1.5 g, PO 6 h after initial dose; alternatively, the parenteral regimen may be repeated 8 h after initial dose
Ampicillin/amoxicillin/penicillin-allergic patients unable to take oral medication	
Vancomycin and gentamicin	IV administration of vancomycin, 1.0 g, over 1 h plus IV or IM administration of gentamicin, 1.5 mg/kg (not to exceed 80 mg), 1 h before procedure; may be repeated once 8 h after initial dose
Alternate low-risk patient regimen	
Amoxicillin	3.0 g PO 1 h before procedure; then 1.5 g 6 h after initial dose

[a]Initial pediatric doses are as follows: ampicillin, 50 mg/kg; amoxicillin, 50 mg/kg; gentamicin, 2.0 mg/kg; and vancomycin, 20 mg/kg. Follow-up doses should be one-half the initial dose. *Total pediatric dose should not exceed total adult dose.*

PROPHYLAXIS FOR MEDICAL CONDITIONS

Indication	Drug and Dosage	Comments
Haemophilus influenzae meningitis exposure	Rifampin 20 mg/kg PO qd x 4 doses (maximum 600 mg/day)	Day care and household contact
Herpes genitalis recurrent	Acyclovir 200 mg PO tid to qid	Use in those with frequent recurrences. May be continued for 18-24 months.
Influenza due to type A influenza	Amantadine 100 mg PO qd x 5-7 weeks	Use as supplement or in addition to vaccine in those at high risk: elderly persons, those with chronic disease, health care providers
Meningococcal exposure	Rifampin 600 mg q12h x 4 doses Children: 10 mg/kg q12h x 4	Only for close (family) contact
Pertussis exposure	Erythromycin 50 mg/kg/day in 4 divided doses for 14 hours	Household or other close contacts
Pneumocystis carinii in AIDS patients	Trimethoprim/sulfamethoxazole or Pentamidine aerosolized	Institute after first episode of *Pneumocystis carinii* or if CD-4 cells fall below 200

Post-splenectomy	Benzathine penicillin G 1.2 million U IM q month for 2-3 years	Patients should receive pneumococcal polyvalent, *Haemophilus influenza* type B, and meningococcal vaccines (prior to splenectomy best)
Prevention of rheumatic fever recurrence	Benzathine penicillin G 1.2 million U IM q month, or Penicillin G or V 200,000 U PO qd, or Sulfadiazine 1.0 g PO qd	Usually started after first episode of rheumatic fever and continued until age 40-50
Prevention of traveler's diarrhea	Trimethoprim/sulfamethoxazole Doxycycline Norfloxacin Ciprofloxacin Bismuth subsalicylate	Not recommended for general usage, but all have proven efficacy

Section 7

ANTIMICROBIAL AGENTS IN PREGNANCY

May be Harmful Generally Contradicated	Try to Avoid Use Only if Essential	Probably Safe, Use When Clearly Indicated
Amantadine	Acyclovir	Amoxicillin
Cinoxacin	Amikacin	Amoxicillin/clavulanate
Ciprofloxacin	Aminoglycosides	Ampicillin
Colistin sulfate	Aminosalicylic acid	Azlocillin
Dehydroemetine	Amphotericin B	Aztreonam
Doxycycline[a]		
Emetine	Capreomycin	Bacampicillin
Flucytosine	Chloramphenicol[b]	Carbenicillin
Ganciclovir	Clindamycin	Cefadroxil
Griseofulvin	Cotrimoxazole	Cefamandole
Nalidixic acid	Cycloserine	Cefazolin
Norfloxacin		Cefonicid
Ofloxacin	Erythromycin estolate	Cefotaxime
Primaquine	Ethambutol	Cefotetan
Quinolones	Ethionamide	Cefoxitin
Ribavirin	Fluconazole	
Tetracycline[a]	Gentamicin	Ceftazidime
Tetracyclines[a]	Itraconazole	Ceftizoxime
	Kanamycin	Ceftriaxone
	Ketoconazole	Cefuroxime
	Lincomycin	Cephalexin
	Mebendazole	Cephalosporins
		Cephalothin
	Metronidazole	Cephapirin
		Cephradine
	Moxalactam	Cloxacillin
	Netilmicin	Cyclacillin
	Niclosamide	Dicloxacillin
	Nitrofurantoin[b]	Erythromycin (not estolate)
		Imipenem/cilastatin

May be Harmful Generally Contradicated	Try to Avoid Use Only if Essential	Probably Safe, Use When Clearly Indicated
	Pentamidine	
		Isoniazid
		Methenamine hippurate
	Praziquantel	Methenamine mandelate
	Pyrantel	Methicillin
	Pyrazinamide	
	Pyrimethamine	Mezlocillin
	Quinacrine	Nafcillin
		Nystatin
	Quinine	Oxacillin
		Penicillins
	Spectinomycin	Piperacillin
	Streptomycin	Piperazine
		Rifampin
	Sulfonamides[b]	Ticarcillin
		Ticarcillin/clavulanate
	Thiabendazole	
	Tobramycin	
	Trimethoprim	
	Trimethoprim/sulfamethoxazole[b]	
	Vancomycin	
	Vidarabrine	
	Zidovudine	

[a]Contraindicated in last half of pregnancy, IV use contraindicated, prolonged therapy contraindicated.
[b]Contraindicated at term.
(Adapted from Safety of Antimicrobial Agents in Pregnancy. Med Let 29:61–63, 1987, with permission).

Section 8

PHARMACOLOGY AND DOSAGE OF ANTIMICROBIAL AGENTS

Drug	Dosage Recommendations		
	Adults		Children
	Dose/Interval	Daily Dose for Serious Infection	Dose/Interval
Acyclovir	0.2-0.8 g q4h (5 doses/ day) PO	2.0-3.0 g	
	5-10 mg/kg q8h IV	30 mg/kg	5-15 mg/kg q8h IV
Amantadine	0.1 g q12h or 0.1-0.2 g q24h PO	0.2 g	2.2-4.4 mg/kg q12h PO
Amikacin	5 mg/kg q8h or 7.5 mg/kg q12h IV/IM	15 mg/kg	5 mg/kg q8h or 7.5 mg/kg q12h IV/IM
Amoxicillin	0.25-0.5 g q8h PO	1.5 g	6.6-13.3 mg/kg q8h PO
Amoxicillin + clavulanate	0.25-0.5 g q8h PO	1.5 g	6.6-13.3 mg/kg q8h PO
Amphotericin	0.25-1 mg/kg q24h IV	0.6 mg/kg	0.25-1 mg/kg q24h IV
Ampicillin	0.5-1 g q6h PO	4 g	12.5-25 mg/kg q6h PO
	1-2 g q4-6h IV/IM	8-12 g	25-50 mg/kg q6h IV/IM
Ampicillin + sulbactam	0.5-1 g q6h PO 1.5-3.0 g q6h IV/IM	4 g 8-12 g	12.5-25 mg/kg q6h PO 25-50 mg/kg q6h IV/IM
Azlocillin	2-4 g q4-6h IV/IM	18-24 g	50 mg/kg q4h or 75 mg/kg q6h (not approved) IV/IM
Aztreonam	0.5-2 g q6-12h IV/IM	6-8 g	18.75-37.5 mg/kg q6h IV/IM (not approved)
Bacampicillin	0.4-0.8 g q12h PO	1.6 g	12.5-25 mg/kg q12h PO
Capreomycin	0.75-1 g q24h	1 g	15-30 mg/kg/day IM (not approved)
Carbenicillin	5-6.5 g q4-6h IV/IM	24-30 g	25-100 mg/kg q4-6h IV/IM

| | Usual Adult Dose and Interval Adjustment | | | | Dosage for Dialysis | |
| | For Creatinine Clearance (ml/min) | | | | | |
Dose	>80	80-50	50-10	<10 (Anuric)	Dose After HD Supplemental to Anuric	Daily Dose During PD
5 mg/kg	8 hr	8 hr	12-24 hr	2.5 mg/kg q24h	Give daily dose after HD	
200 mg q24h or 100 mg q12h PO	12 hr	100 mg q12-24h	200 mg/day alternate days to alternating q7 days	200 mg/day alternate days to alternating q7 days	None	
5-7.5 mg/kg	8-12 hr	12 hr	24-36 hr	36-48 hr	2.5-3.75 mg/kg	3-4 mg/2 L dialysate removed
0.25-0.5 g PO	8 hr	8 hr	12 hr	12-24 hr	0.25 g	
0.25-0.5 g PO	8 hr	8 hr	12 hr	12-24 hr	0.25 g	
0.25-1 mg/kg IV	24 hr	24 hr	24 hr	24 hr	No change	
1-2 g	4-6 hr	6 hr	8 hr	12 hr	0.5 g	
1-2 g	4-6 hr	6 hr	8 hr	12 hr	0.5 g	
2-4 g	4-6 hr	4-6 hr	8 hr	12 hr	3 g	
0.5-2 g	6-12 hr	8-12 hr	12-24 hr	24-36 hr	15 mg/kg	30 mg/kg q24h
0.4-0.8 g PO	12 hr	12 hr	12 hr	24 hr		
0.75-1 g	24 hr					
5-6.5 g	4-6 hr	6 hr	2-3 g q6-8h	2 g q12h	2 g	2 g q6h

(Continues)

Drug	Dosage Recommendations		
	Adults		Children
	Dose/Interval	Daily Dose for Serious Infection	Dose/Interval
Carbenicillin indanyl sodium	1-2 tablets (382 mg each) q6h PO	3 g	7.5-12.5 mg/kg q6h PO
Cefaclor	0.25-0.5 g q8h PO	1.5 g	6.6-13.3 mg/kg q8h PO
Cefadroxil	1-2 g/day q12-24h PO	2 g	15 mg/kg q12h PO
Cefamandole	1-2 g q4-6h IV/IM	4-8 g	50-150 mg/kg/day q4-8h IV/IM
Cefazolin	0.5-1.5 g q6-8h IV/IM	3-6 g	8.3-25 mg/kg q6-8h IV/IM
Cefixime	0.4 g/day q12-24h PO	0.4 g	8 mg/kg/day as q12-24h PO
Cefmenoxime	0.5-2 g q4-6h IV/IM	8 g	10-20 mg/kg q6h IV/IM
Cefmetazole	2 g q6-8h IV	8 g	
Cefonicid	0.5-2 g q24h IV/IM	2 g	
Ceforanide	0.5-1 g q12h IV/IM	1-2 g	10-20 mg/kg q12h IV
Cefoperazone	1-4 g q8h or 0.5-3 g q6h IV/IM	6-12 g	25-100 mg/kg q12h IV/IM
Cefotaxime	1-2 g q4-12h IV/IM	6-12 g	50-180 mg/kg/day as q4-6h IV/IM
Cefotetan	1-2 g q12h IV/IM	4 g	20-30 mg/kg q8-12h IV/IM

| | Usual Adult Dose and Interval Adjustment | | | | Dosage for Dialysis | |
| | For Creatinine Clearance (ml/min) | | | | | |
Dose	>80	80-50	50-10	<10 (Anuric)	Dose After HD Supplemental to Anuric	Daily Dose During PD
0.25-0.5 g PO	8 hr	8 hr	8 hr (50-100% usual dose)	8 hr (25-33% usual dose)	Repeat dose after HD	
1 g PO	12-24 hr	12-24 hr	25-50: q12h 10-25: q24h	36-48 hr	0.5-1 g	
0.5-2 g	4-6 hr	1-2 g q6h	1-2 g q8h	0.5-1 g q12h	Supplemental dose	No supplemental dose
0.5-1.5 g	6-8 hr	8 hr	0.5-1 g q8-12h	0.5-1 g q24h	0.25-0.5 g	
				0.2 g q24h	No supplemental dose	No supplemental dose
0.5-2 g	4-6 hr	6-8 hr	12-24 hr	24 hr	30-50% maintenance dose	
2 g	8 hr	8 hr	16 hr	48 hr		
0.5-2 g	24 hr	0.5-1.5 g q24h	0.25-1 g q24-48h	0.25-1 g q3-5d	No extra dose	
1-4 g	6-8 hr	6-8 hr	6-8 hr	6-8 hr	Schedule the dose after dialysis	
1-2 g	4-8 hr	4-8 hr	6-12 hr	12 hr	Maintenance dose x 50%	
1-2 g	12 hr	12 hr	24 hr	48 hr	Supplemental dose	

(Continues)

Drug	Dosage Recommendations		
	Adults		Children
	Dose/Interval	Daily Dose for Serious Infection	Dose/Interval
Cefoxitin	1-2 g q4-6h or 3 g q6h IV/IM	4-8 g	20-26.6 mg/kg q4-6h IM/IV
Cefpiramide	1-4 g q12-24h IV/IM	4 g	
Cefpirome	1-2 g q12h IV/IM	4 g	
Cefsulodin	1-2 g q6-8h IV/IM	6 g	15-25 mg/kg q6h IV/IM
Ceftazidime	0.5-2 g q8-12h IV/IM	6 g	30-50 mg/kg q8h IV/IM
Ceftizoxime	1-4 g q8-12h IV/IM	6-12 g	50 mg/kg q6-8h IV/IM
Ceftriaxone	.1-2 g q12-24h IV/IM	2 g	50-75 mg/kg/day as q12-24h IV/IM, 50 mg/kg q12h for meningitis
Cefuroxime	0.75-1.5 g q8h IV/IM	4.5 g	50-240 mg/kg/day as q6-8h IV/IM
Cefuroxime axetil	0.125-0.5 g q12h PO	0.5-1 g	0.125-0.5 g q12h PO
Cephalexin	0.25-1 g q6h PO	2 g	6.25-25 mg/kg q6h PO
Cephalothin	0.5-2 g q4-6h IV	6-12 g	75-160 mg/kg/day as q4-6h IV/IM
Cephapirin	0.5-2 g q4-6h IV	6-12 g	10-20 mg/kg q6h IV/IM

| | Usual Adult Dose and Interval Adjustment | | | | Dosage for Dialysis | |
| | For Creatinine Clearance (ml/min) | | | | | |
Dose	>80	80-50	50-10	<10 (Anuric)	Dose After HD Supplemental to Anuric	Daily Dose During PD
1-3 g	4-6 hr	1-2 g q8h	1-2 g q12h	0.5-1 g q12-24h	1-2 g	
0.5-3 g	6 hr	8 hr	0.25-1.5 g q6h or 1 g q12h	0.5 g q12h or 1 g q24h	0.25 g	1 g q18-24h
0.5-2 g	8-12 hr	8-12 hr	1-1.5 g q12-24h	0.5-0.75 g q24-48h	1 g loading 1 g post dialysis	1 g then 0.5 g q24h
1-4 g	8-12 hr	0.5-1.5 g q8h	0.25-1 g q12h	0.25-1 g q24-48h	Give scheduled dose after dialysis	3 g q48h
0.5-1 g	12-24 hr	12-24 hr	12-24 hr	12-24 hr	No supplemental dose	
0.75-1.5 g	8 hr	8 hr	8-12 hr	24 hr	Supplemental dose	No supplemental dose
0.25-1 g PO	6 hr	6 hr	500 mg 8-12 hr	250 mg q12-24h	0.25-1 g	
0.5-2 g	4-6 hr	6 hr	8 hr	0.5 g q6-8h	Supplemental dose	No supplemental dose
0.5-2 g	4-6 hr	6 hr	8 hr	12 hr	7.5-15 mg/kg before dialysis	

(Continues)

Drug	Dosage Recommendations		
	Adults		Children
	Dose/Interval	Daily Dose for Serious Infection	Dose/Interval
Cephradine	0.25-1 g q6-12h PO	2 g	6.25-12.5 mg/kg q6-12h PO
	0.5-2 g q6h IV/IM	4-8 g	12.5-25 mg/kg q6h IV/IM
Chloramphenicol	12.5-25 mg/kg q6h PO	4 g	12.5-25 mg/kg q6h PO
	12.5-25 mg/kg q6h IV/IM	4 g	12.5-25 mg/kg q6h IV/IM
Chlortetracycline	0.25-0.5 g q6h PO	2 g	25-50 mg/kg/day as q6h PO
Ciprofloxacin	0.25-0.75 g q12h PO	1.5 g	Not recommended
	0.2-0.4 g q12h IV	0.8 g	
Clarithromycin	0.25-0.5 g q12h PO	1 g	
Clindamycin	0.15-0.45 g q6h PO	1.2 g	2-8 mg/kg q6-8h PO
	0.15-0.9 g q6-8h IV/IM	1.8-2.7 g	2.5-10 mg/kg q6h IV/IM
Clofazimine	0.1 g/day PO	0.1 g	
Cloxacillin	0.5-1 g q6h PO	2 g	12.5-25 mg/kg q6h PO
Colistimethate	0.8-1.7 mg/kg q8h IV/IM	5 mg/kg	1.7-2.3 mg/kg q8h IV/IM
Cotrimoxazole	2 tablets q12h or 1 tablet q6h PO (each tablet = 80 mg trimethoprim and 400 mg sulfamethoxazole; 1 double-strength (DS) tablet = 160/800 mg)	4 tablets PO	4-5 mg/kg q6-12h (as TMP) PO
	4-5 mg/kg q6-12h (as TMP) IV	1.2 g TMP, 6 g SMX IV	4-5 mg/kg q6-12h (as TMP) IV

| | Usual Adult Dose and Interval Adjustment | | | | Dosage for Dialysis | |
| | For Creatinine Clearance (ml/min) | | | | | |
Dose	>80	80-50	50-10	<10 (Anuric)	Dose After HD Supplemental to Anuric	Daily Dose During PD
1-2 g	6 hr	6 hr	8 h or 250-500 mg q6h	250 mg q12-24h	1-2 g	500 mg q6h for CAPD
12.5-25 mg/kg	6 hr	6 hr	6 hr	6 hr	Schedule the dose after dialysis	No change
0.25-0.5 g PO	6 hr	Not recommended	Not recommended	Not recommended		
0.25-0.75	12 hr	12 hr	0.25-0.5 g 12-18 hr	0.25-0.5 g 24 hr	Give 0.25-0.5 g q24h after dialysis	
0.25-0.5 g	12 hr	12 hr	Decrease dose			
0.15-0.9 g	6-8 hr	6-8 hr	6-8 hr	6-8 hr	None	No change
0.1 g PO	24 hr					
0.5-1 g PO	6 hr	6 hr	6 hr	6 hr		
0.8-1.7 mg/kg	8 hr	2.5 mg/kg on day 1, then 1-1.5 mg/kg q24h	2.5 mg/kg on day 1, then 1-1.5 mg/kg q24-72h	2.5 mg/kg on day 1, then 1-1.5 mg/kg q48-72h		
4-5 mg/kg (as TMP)	6-12 hr	12 hr	18 hr	24-48 hr	4-5 mg/kg (as TMP)	0.16/0.8 q48h

(Continues)

Drug	Dosage Recommendations		
	Adults		Children
	Dose/Interval	Daily Dose for Serious Infection	Dose/Interval
Cycloserine	0.25-0.5 g q12h PO	1 g	3.5-5 mg/kg q12h PO (not approved)
Dapsone	100 mg/day	100 mg/day	25-100 mg/day
Demeclocycline	0.15 g q6h or 0.3 g q12h PO	0.6 g	6.6-13.2 mg/kg/day as q6-12h PO
Dicloxacillin	0.25-0.5 g q6h PO	2 g	3.125-6.25 mg/kg q6h PO
Didanosine	300 mg q12h (two 150 mg tablets) PO for body weight >75 kg 200 mg q12h (two 100 mg tablet) PO for body weight 50-74 kg 125 mg q12h (one 100 mg and one 25 mg tablets) PO for body weight 35-49 kg		100 mg q12h (two 50 mg tablets) PO for body surface 1.1-1.4 M^2 75 mg q12h (one 50 mg and one 25 mg tablet) PO for body surface 0.8-1.1 M^2 50 mg q12h (two 25 mg tablets) PO for body suface 0.5-0.7 M^2 25 mg q12h (one 25 mg tablet) PO for body surface <0.4 M^2
Doxycycline	0.1 g q12-24h PO	0.2 g	2.2 mg/kg q12-24h PO
	0.1 g q12-24h IV/IM	0.2 g	2.2 mg/kg q12-24h IV/IM
Erythromycin	0.25-0.5 g q6h PO	2 g	7.5-12.5 mg/kg q6h PO
	0.25-1 g q6h IV	4 g	3.75-12.5 mg/kg q6h IV/IM
Erythromycin base	0.333 g q8h PO	2 g	7.5-12.5 mg/kg q6h PO
stearate	0.25-0.5 g q6-12h PO	2 g	
ethyl succinate	0.4 g q6-12h PO	2 g	
Erythromycin estolate	0.25-0.5 g q6-12h PO	2 g	40 mg/kg/day as q6-12h PO

Dose	>80	80-50	50-10	<10 (Anuric)	Dose After HD Supplemental to Anuric	Daily Dose During PD
		Usual Adult Dose and Interval Adjustment			**Dosage for Dialysis**	
		For Creatinine Clearance (ml/min)				
0.25-0.5 g PO	12 hr					
Not known					Not known	Not known
0.15-0.3 g PO	6-12 hr	Not recommended	Not recommended	Not recommended		
0.25-0.5 g PO	6 hr	6 hr	6 hr	6 hr		
As before by body weight or surface area	Unchanged	Reduction advised	Reduction advised	Reduction advised		
0.1 g PO	12-24 hr	12-24 hr	12-24 hr	12-24 hr	No supplemental dose	No supplemental dose
0.25-1 g	6 hr	6 hr	6 hr	6 hr	None	No change
0.25-1 g	6 hr	6 hr	6 hr	6 hr	None	No change
0.25-1 g	6 hr	6 hr	6 hr	6 hr	None	No change

(Continues)

Drug	Dosage Recommendations		
	Adults		Children
	Dose/Interval	Daily Dose for Serious Infection	Dose/Interval
Erythromycin gluceptate	0.25-0.5 g IV q6h	4 g	30-50 mg/kg/day as q6h IM
Erythromycin lactobionate	0.25-0.5 g IV q6h	4 g	30-50 mg/kg/day q6h IM
Ethambutol	15 mg/kg q24h PO	15 mg/kg/day	15 mg/kg q24h PO (not approved)
Ethionamide	0.25-0.5 g q12h PO	1 g	5-10 mg/kg q12h PO (not approved)
Fluconazole	0.2-0.4 g q24h PO	0.4 g	
	0.2-0.4 g q24h IV	0.4 g	
Flucytosine	37.5 mg/kg q6h PO	150 mg/kg	37.5 mg/kg q6h PO
	37.5 mg/kg q6h IV	150 mg/kg	
Foscarnet	60 mg/kg q8h for 14 days for induction	180 mg/kg	
	90 mg/kg/day IV for maintenance	90 mg/kg	
Ganciclovir	5 mg/kg IV q12h	5 mg/kg qd maintenance	10 mg/kg; 5 mg/kg maintenance
Gentamicin	1-1.7 mg/kg q8h IV/IM	3-5 mg/kg	1-2.5 mg/kg q8h IV/IM
Griseofulvin	0.5-1 g/day in single or 2-4 doses PO	1 g	10 mg/kg/day PO
Hetacillin	0.225-0.45 g q6h PO	1.8 g	5.6-11.25 mg/kg q6h PO
Imipenem	0.5-1 g q6-8h IV/IM	2 g	15-25 mg/kg q6h IV/IM

| | Usual Adult Dose and Interval Adjustment | | | | Dosage for Dialysis | |
| | For Creatinine Clearance (ml/min) | | | | | |
Dose	>80	80-50	50-10	<10 (Anuric)	Dose After HD Supplemental to Anuric	Daily Dose During PD
0.25-1 g	6 hr	6 hr	6 hr	6 hr	None	No change
0.25-1 g	6 hr	6 hr	6 hr	6 hr	None	No change
15 mg/kg PO	24 hr	24 hr	48 hr	72 hr	15 mg/kg on dialysis day	15 mg/kg/day during PD
0.25-0.5 g PO	12 hr	12 hr	12 hr	24 hr		
0.2-0.4 g PO	24 hr	24 hr	48 hr	$\geq$72 hr		
37.5 mg/kg PO	6 hr	6 hr	12-24 hr	15-25 mg/kg q24h or by plasma level of 50-75	20-37.5 mg/kg	
90 mg/kg /day IV (maintenance)	90 mg/kg/day	75 mg/kg/day	63-71 mg/kg/day	57 mg/kg/day		
5 mg/kg	12 hr	12 hr	24 hr	24 hr	5 mg/kg	
1.5 mg/kg	8 hr	8-12 hr	12-24 hr	24-48 hr	1-1.5 mg/kg	1 mg/2 L dialysate removed
0.5-1 g PO	24 hr	24 hr	24 hr	24 hr		
1-2 g	4-6 hr	6 hr	8 hr	12 hr	0.5 g	
0.5-1 g	6-8 hr	0.5 g q6-8h	0.5 g q6-12h	0.25-0.5 g q24h	2 g/day max and 1 dose after HD	

(Continues)

Drug	Dosage Recommendations		
	Adults		Children
	Dose/Interval	Daily Dose for Serious Infection	Dose/Interval
Interferon-α hepatitis B	5 million U subcutaneously qd for 4 months		Not known
hepatitis C	2-3 million U subcutaneously tiw for 6 months		Not known
Isoniazid	5 mg/kg/day (0.3 g) PO	0.3 g	10-20 mg/kg/day as q12-24h PO
	5 mg/kg/day IM	0.3 g	10-20 mg/kg/day as q12-24h IM
Itraconazole	0.2-0.4 g q24h PO	0.4 g	
Kanamycin	5 mg/kg q8h or 7.5 mg/kg q12h IM or IV	1.5 g	5 mg/kg q8h IM or IV
Ketoconazole	0.2-0.4 g q24h PO	0.4 g	5-10 mg/kg/day as q12-24h PO
Methenamine hippurate	1 g q12h PO	2 g	12.5-25 mg/kg q12h PO
Methenamine mandelate	1 g q6h PO	4 g	12.5-18.75 mg/kg q6h PO
Methicillin	1-2 g q4-6h IV/IM	12 g	25-33.3 mg/kg q4-6h IV/IM
Metronidazole	7.5 mg/kg q6h PO	30 mg/kg	7.5 mg/kg q6h PO
	7.5 mg/kg q6h IV/IM	30 mg/kg	7.5 mg/kg q6h IV/IM
Mezlocillin	3-4 g q4-6h IV/IM	18-24 g	50 mg/kg q4-6h IV/IM
Miconazole	0.6-1.2 g q8h IV	1.8-3.6 g	6.6-13.3 mg/kg q8h IV
Minocycline	0.2 g once then 0.1 g q12h PO	0.2 g	4 mg/kg once then 2 mg/kg q12h PO
	0.2 g once then 0.1 g q12h IV/IM	0.2 g	4 mg/kg once then 2 mg/kg q12h IV/IM

| | Usual Adult Dose and Interval Adjustment | | | | Dosage for Dialysis | |
| | For Creatinine Clearance (ml/min) | | | | | |
Dose	>80	80-50	50-10	<10 (Anuric)	Dose After HD Supplemental to Anuric	Daily Dose During PD
5 mg/kg PO	24 hr	24 hr	24 hr	24 hr	5 mg/kg	
0.2-0.4 g PO	24 hr	24 hr	24 hr	24 hr		
5-7.5 mg/kg	8-12 hr	24 hr	24-72 hr	72-96 hr	5 mg/kg	3.75 mg/kg qd
0.2-0.4 g PO	24 hr	24 hr	24 hr	24 hr		
1 g PO	12 hr	12 hr	Not recom-mended	Not recom-mended		
1 g PO	6 hr	6 hr	Not recom-mended	Not recom-mended		
1-2 g	4-6 hr	6 hr	8 hr	12 hr	2 g	
7.5 mg/kg	6 hr	6 hr	6 hr	6 hr	No change	No change
3-4 g	4-6 hr	4-6 hr	6-8 hr	8-12 hr	2-3 g	Anuric dosage
0.6-1.2 g IV	8 hr	8 hr	8 hr	8 hr		
0.1 g PO	6-12 hr	Not recom-mended	Not recom-mended	Not recom-mended		

(Continues)

Drug	Dosage Recommendations		
	Adults		Children
	Dose/Interval	Daily Dose for Serious Infection	Dose/Interval
Moxalactam	0.5-4 g q8-12h IV/IM	8 g	50 mg/kg q6-8h IV/IM
Nafcillin	0.5-1 g q6h PO	2 g	12.5-25 mg/kg q6h PO
	0.5-1.5 g q4-6h IV/IM	9 g	150 mg/kg/day as q4-6h IV/IM
Nalidixic acid	1 g q6h PO	4 g	Not recommended
Neomycin	6.6 mg/kg q4h $\leq$3 days PO	3 g PO	12.5-25 mg/kg q6h PO
Netilmicin	1.5-3.25 mg/kg q12h or 1.3-2.2 mg/kg q8h IM	3.9 mg/kg	1-2.5 mg/kg q8h IM
Nitrofurantoin	0.05-0.1 g q6h PO	0.4 g	1.25-1.75 mg/kg q6h PO
Norfloxacin	0.2-0.4 g q12h PO	0.8 g	
Nystatin	400,000-600,000 U q6h (4-6 ml) PO	2 million U	250,000-500,000 U q6h (2.5-5 ml) PO
Ofloxacin	0.2-0.4 g q12h PO	0.8 g	Not recommended
Oxacillin	0.5-1 g q6h PO	4 g	12.5-25 mg/kg q6h PO
	0.5-2 g q4-6h IV/IM	6-12 g	37.5-50 mg/kg q6h IV/IM
Oxolinic acid	0.75 q12h PO	1.5 g	Not recommended
Oxytetracycline	0.25-0.5 g q6h PO	2 g	25-50 mg/kg/day as q6-12h PO
	0.25-0.5 g q12h IV	2 g	6 mg/kg q12h IV
Para-amino salicylic acid	3 g q6-8h PO	12 g	66.6-75 mg/kg q6-8h PO
Penicillin G	0.5-1 g q6h PO	2-4 g	6.25-12.5 mg/kg q6h PO
	1.2-24 x 10^6 U/day as q2-12h IV	24 x 10^6 U	100,000-250,000 U/kg/day q2-12h IV

| | Usual Adult Dose and Interval Adjustment | | | | Dosage for Dialysis | |
| | For Creatinine Clearance (ml/min) | | | | | |
Dose	>80	80-50	50-10	<10 (Anuric)	Dose After HD Supplemental to Anuric	Daily Dose During PD
0.5-4 g	8-12 hr	0.5-3 g q8h	0.25-2 g q8h or 0.25-3 g q12h	0.25 g q12h to 1 g q24h	1-2 g	1 g q36-48h or 0.5g q18-24h
0.5-1.5 g	4-6 hr	4-6 hr	4-6 hr	4-6 hr		
1 g PO	6 hr	6 hr	6 hr	Not recommended		
6.6 mg/kg PO	4 hr					
1.3•2.2 mg/kg	8 hr	8-12 hr	12-24 hr	24-48 hr	2 mg/kg	
0.05-0.1 g PO	6 hr	6 hr	Not recommended	Not recommended		
0.2-0.4 g PO	12 hr	12 hr	12-24 hr	24 hr		
400,000-600,000 U PO	6 hr	6 hr	6 hr	6 hr		
0.2	12 hr	12 hr	24-48 hr	48 hr	None	
0.5-2 g	4-6 hr	4-6 hr	4-6 hr	4-6 hr		
0.75 g PO	12 hr		Not recommended	Not recommended		
0.25-0.5 g PO	6 hr	Not recommended	Not recommended	Not recommended		
3 g PO	6-8 hr					
1.2-24 x 10^6 U	2-12 hr	2-12 hr	2-12 hr	⅓-½ maximum daily dose	0.5 x 10^6 U	

(Continues)

Drug	Dosage Recommendations		
	Adults		Children
	Dose/Interval	Daily Dose for Serious Infection	Dose/Interval
Penicillin G benzathine	$0.6\text{-}2.4 \times 10^6$ U IM g once or weekly x 3	$1.2\text{-}2.4 \times 10^6$ U IM	50,000 U/kg IM
Penicillin G procaine	$0.3\text{-}4.8 \times 10^6$ U IM q12-24h	1.2-4.8 g	25,000 U/kg q12-24h
Penicillin V (phenoxymethyl penicillin)	0.25-0.5 g q6h PO	2 g	6.25-12.5 mg/kg q6h PO
Piperacillin	3-4 g q4-6h IV/IM	18 g	50 mg/kg q4-6h (not approved) IV/IM
Pyrazinamide	15-30 mg/kg/day PO in 2-4 divided doses	2 g	15-30 mg/kg/day PO in 2-4 divided doses
Quinidine gluconate	10 mg/kg over 1-2 hr followed by 0.02 mg/kg/min IV	—	10 mg/kg over 1-2 hr followed by 0.02 mg/kg/min IV
Ribavirin			Aerosol 190 µg/L at 12.5 L/min over 12-18 hr/day
Rifabutin	0.15-0.3 g/day PO	0.3 g	
Rifampin	0.6 g/24 hr PO	0.6 g	10-20 mg/kg/day as q12-24h PO
	0.3-0.6 g/day IV	0.6 mg/day IV	10-20 mg/kg/day IV not to exceed 600 mg
Rimantadine	0.1 g q12-24h PO	0.2 g	3 mg/kg q12h PO
Roxithromycin	0.15 g q12h or 0.3 g q24h PO		2.5-5 mg/kg q12h PO
Spectinomycin	2 g once IM	2 g	40 mg/kg once IM
Streptomycin	7.5-15 mg/kg/day IM	1 g	10-15 mg/kg q12h IM
Sulfadiazine	2-4 g initial dose, then 0.5-1 g q4-6h PO	4 g	120-750 mg/kg/day as q4-6h PO
Sulfadoxine-pyrimethamine	1 tablet every wk or 2 tablets every other wk (each tablet = 500 mg sulfadoxine and 25 mg pyrimethamine) (prophylaxis)		By age PO (see *PPID*, p. 408)

	Usual Adult Dose and Interval Adjustment				Dosage for Dialysis	
	For Creatinine Clearance (ml/min)					
Dose	>80	80-50	50-10	<10 (Anuric)	Dose After HD Supplemental to Anuric	Daily Dose During PD
	No change necessary					
	No change necessary					
0.25-0.5 g PO	6 hr	6 hr	8 hr	12 hr	0.25 g	
3-4 g	4-6 hr	4-6 hr	6-12 hr	12 hr	2 g q8h + 1 g after HD	
25 mg/kg/day PO	6-12 hr					
			Not known	Not known	Not known	Not known
0.15-0.3 g PO	24 hr	24 hr	0.15 g q24h	0.075 g q72h		
0.6 g PO	24 hr	24 hr	24 hr	24 hr	No supplemental dose	No supplemental dose
0.6 g IV	24 hr	24 hr	24 hr	24 hr	No supplemental dose	No supplemental dose
0.1 g	4 hr	24 hr	24 hr	24 hr	None	
2 g once						
15 mg/kg/day	24 hr	24 hr	24-72 hr	72-96 hr	5 mg/kg	
0.5-1 g PO	4-6 hr					
0.5 g PO or 1 g PO	every wk or every other wk					

(Continues)

Drug	Dosage Recommendations		
	Adults		Children
	Dose/Interval	Daily Dose for Serious Infection	Dose/Interval
Sulfamethoxazole	1 g q8-12h PO	2 g	25-30 mg/kg q12h PO
Sulfisoxazole	0.5-1 g q6h PO	4 g	120-150 mg/kg/day as q4-6h PO
	25 mg/kg q6h IV	4 g	100 mg/kg/day as q6-8h IV
Tetracycline	0.25-0.5 g q6h PO	2 g	25-50 mg/kg/day as q6-12h PO
	0.125-0.5 g q6-12h IV	2 g	10-20 mg/kg/day as q6-12h IV
Ticarcillin	3 g q4-6h IV/IM	18 g	50 mg/kg q4-6h IV/IM
Ticarcillin + clavulanate	3.1 g q4-8h IV	18.6 g	50 mg/kg q4-6h IV/IM
Tobramycin	1-1.7 mg/kg q8h IV/IM	3 mg/kg	1-2 mg/kg q8h IV/IM
Trimethoprim	0.1 g q12h PO	0.2	2 mg/kg q12h PO (not approved in children <12 years old)
Trimethoprim-sulfamethoxazole (TMP-SMX)	2 tablets q12h or 1 tablet q6h PO (each tablet = 80 mg trimethoprim and 400 mg sulfamethoxazole; 1 double-strength (DS) tablet = 160/800 mg)	4 tablets PO	4-5 mg/kg q6-12h (as TMP) PO
	4-5 mg/kg q6-12h (as TMP) IV	1.2 g TMP, 6 g SMX IV	4-5 mg/kg q6-12h (as TMP) IV
Vancomycin	0.125-0.5 g q6h PO	1 g	12.5 mg/kg q6h PO
	15 mg/kg q12h or 6.5-8 mg/kg q6h IV	2 g	10 mg/kg q6h IV
Vidarabine	10-15 mg/kg/day over 12 hr IV	15 mg/kg	10-15 mg/kg/day over 12 hr IV
Viomycin	1 g q12h twice weekly IV/IM	2 g	
Zidovudine	0.1-0.2 g q4h PO (5 doses)	0.5	80-120 mg/m^2 PO g 4h

	Usual Adult Dose and Interval Adjustment For Creatinine Clearance (ml/min)				Dosage for Dialysis	
Dose	>80	80-50	50-10	<10 (Anuric)	Dose After HD Supplemental to Anuric	Daily Dose During PD
1 g PO	8-12 hr					
0.5-1 g PO	6 hr	6-8 hr	8-12 hr	12-24 hr		
0.25-0.5 g PO	6 hr	Not recommended	Not recommended	Not recommended		
3 g	4-6 hr	4-6 hr	2-3 g q6-8h	2 g q12h	3 g	3 g q12h
3.1 g	4-6 hr	4-6 hr	2-3.1 g q6-8h	2 g q12h	3.1 g	3.1 g q12h
1.5 mg/kg	8 hr	8-12 hr	12-24 hr	24-48 hr	1 mg/kg	1 mg/2 L dialysate removed
0.1 g PO	12 hr	12 hr	24 hr	24-48 hr		
4-5 mg/kg (as TMP)	6-12 hr	12 hr	18 hr	24-48 hr	4-5 mg/kg (as TMP)	0.16/0.8 q48h
15 mg/kg q12h or 6.5-8 mg/kg q6h	6-12 hr	See *Principles and Practice of Infectious Diseases*, 3rd Ed., Ch. 27			No change	
10-15 mg/kg/day	10-15 mg/kg/day	10-15 mg/kg/day	10-15 mg/kg/day	7.5-15 mg/kg/day	Give daily dose after HD	
1 g	12 hr twice weekly					
100 mg	4 hr	4 hr	4 hr	4 hr		

Section 9

GENERIC/TRADE AND TRADE/GENERIC LISTS

Generic	Trade	Family
Acyclovir	Zovirax	Antiviral agents
Albendazole	Zentel	Antiparasitic agents
Amantadine	Symmetrel	Antiviral agents
Amdinocillin	Coactin	Penicillins
Amikacin	Amikin	Aminoglycosides
Amithiozone (thiacetazone)	Panthrone Tibione	Antimycobacterials
Amoxicillin	Amoxil Larotid Polymox Robamox Trimox	Penicillins
Amoxicillin + clavulanate	Augmentin	β-Lactamase inhibitors + penicillins
Amphotericin B	Fungizone	Antifungal agents
Ampicillin	Ampen Amcill Omnipen Omnipen N PenA Penbritin Pensyn Polycillin Polycillin N Principen Probampacin Supen Totacillin	Penicillins

Generic	Trade	Family
Ampicillin probenecid	Polycillin-PRB Trojacillin-Plus	Penicillins
Ampicillin + sulbactam	Unasyn	β-Lactamase inhibitors + penicillins
Aspoxicillin	Doyle	Penicillins
Azithromycin	Zithromax	Macrolides
Azlocillin	Azlin	Penicillins
Aztreonam	Azactam	Other β-lactams
Bacampicillin	Spectrobid	Penicillins
Benzathine penicillin	Bicillin Permapen	Penicillins
Bithionol	Bitrin Lorothidol	Antiparasitic agents
Capreomycin	Capastat	Antimycobacterial agents
Carbenicillin	Geopen Pyopen	Penicillins
Carbenicillin indanyl sodium	Geocillin	Penicillins
Cefaclor	Ceclor	Cephalosporins
Cefadroxil	Duricef	Cephalosporins
Cefamandole	Mandol	Cephalosporins
Cefazolin	Ancef Kefzol	Cephalosporins

(Continues)

Generic	Trade	Family
Cefbuperazone	Keiperazon	Cephalosporins
Cefixime	Suprax	Cephalosporins
Cefmenoxime	Cefmax	Cephalosporins
Cefmetazole	Zefazone	Cephalosporins
Cefminox	Meicelin	Cephalosporins
Cefonicid	Monocid	Cephalosporins
Cefoperazone	Cefobid	Cephalosporins
Cefoperazone + sulbactam	Sulperazone	Cephalosporins + β-lactamase inhibitors
Ceforanide	Precef	Cephalosporins
Cefotaxime	Claforan	Cephalosporins
Cefotetan	Apace Cefotan	Cephalosporins
Cefotiam	Pansporin	Cephalosporins
Cefoxitin	Mefoxin	Cephalosporins
Cefpiramide	Suncefal	Cephalosporins
Cefpirome	—	Cephalosporins
Cefsulodin	Cefomonil	Cephalosporins
Ceftazidime	Fortaz Tazicef Tazidime	Cephalosporins
Ceftizoxime	Cefizox	Cephalosporins

Generic	Trade	Family
Ceftriaxone	Rocephin	Cephalosporins
Cefuroxime	Zinacef Kefurox	Cephalosporins
Cefuroxime axetil	Ceftin	Cephalosporins
Cefuzonam	Cosmosin	Cephalosporins
Cephalexin	Keflex	Cephalosporins
Cephaloglycin	Kafocin	Cephalosporins
Cephalothin	Keflin	Cephalosporins
Cephapirin	Cefadyl Cefatrexail	Cephalosporins
Cephradine	Anspor Velosef	Cephalosporins
Chloramphenicol	Chloromycetin	Chloramphenicol
Chloroquine	Aralen	Antiparasitic agents
Chlortetracycline	Aureomycin	Tetracyclines
Ciprofloxacin	Cipro	Quinolones
Clarithromycin	Biaxin	Macrolides
Clindamycin	Cleocin	Lincosamides
Clofazimine	Lamprene	Antimycobacterial agents
Clotrimazole	Mycelex Lotrimin Canesten	Antifungal agents

(Continues)

Generic	Trade	Family
Cloxacillin	Tegopen	Penicillins
Colistimethate	Colymycin M	Polymyxins
Colistin	Colymycin S	Polymyxins
Cotrimoxazole	Bactrim Septra	Sulfonamides + trimethoprim
Cyclacillin	Cyclapen	Penicillins
Cycloserine	Oxamycin Seromycin	Antimycobacterial agents
Dapsone	Avlosulfon	Antimycobacterial agents
Demeclocycline	Declomycin	Tetracyclines
Dibekacin	Panimycin	Aminoglycosides
Dicloxacillin	Dycill Dynapen Pathocil Veracillin	Penicillins
Didanosine (dideoxyinosine [ddI])	Videx	Antiviral agents
Dideoxycytidine (ddC) (see Zalcitabine)	Hivid	Antiviral agents
Diethylcarbamazine	Hetrazan	Antiparasitic agents
Diloxanide furoate	Furamide	Antiparasitic agents
Doxycycline	Doxy II Doxychel Vibramycin	Tetracyclines

Generic	Trade	Family
Erythromycin	A/T/S Benzamycin E-mycin ERYC Erycette Eryderm Erygel Erymax Ery-Tab Ethril ETS - 2% Ilotycin Kesso-mycin Robimycin	Erythromycins
Erythromycin estolate	Ilosone	Erythromycins
Erythromycin ethylsuccinate	E.E.S Ery-Ped	Erythromycins
Erythromycin ethylsuccinate + sulfisoxazole	Pediazole ESP	Erythromycins + sulfonamides
Erythromycin gluceptate	Ilotycin gluceptate	Erythromycins
Erythromycin lactobionate	Erythrocin lactobionate	Erythromycins
Erythromycin stearate	Erythrocin Wyamycin S	Erythromycins
Ethambutol	Myambutol	Antimycobacterial agents

(Continues)

Generic	Trade	Family
Ethionamide	Trecator-SC	Antimycobacterial agents
Flomoxef	Flumarin	Cephalosporins
Flucloxacillin	Floxapen	Penicillins
Fluconazole	Diflucan	Antifungal agents
Flucytosine	Ancobon	Antifungal agents
Foscarnet	Foscavir	Antiviral agents
Fosfomycin	Fosmicin	
Furazolidone	Furoxone	Antiparasitic agents
Ganciclovir	Cytovene	Antivirals
Gentamicin	Garamycin	Aminoglycosides
Griseofulvin	Fulvicin P-G Fulvicin U F Grifulvin V Gris-PEG Grisactin	Antifungal agents
Hetacillin	Versapen Versapen K	Penicillins
Idoxuridine	Dendrid Herplex Stoxil	Antiviral agents
Imipenem + cilastatin	Primaxin	Carbapenems
Interferon-α-2A, recombinant	Roferon-A	Antiviral agents

Generic	Trade	Family
Interferon-α-2B, recombinant	Intron A	Antiviral agents
Interferon-α-N3	Alferon N	Antiviral agents
Iodoquinol (diiodohydroxyquin)	Yodoxin	Antiparasitic agents
Isoniazid	Hyzyd INH Niadox Niconyl Nydrazid	Antimycobacterial agents
Itraconazole	Sporanox	Antifungal agents
Ivermectin	Mectizan	Antiparasitic agents
Kanamycin	Kantrex	Aminoglycosides
Ketoconazole	Nizoral	Antifungal agents
Mafenide	Sulfamylon	Sulfonamides
Mebendazole	Vermox	Antiparasitic agents
Mefloquine	Lariam	Antiparasitic agents
Melarsoprol B	Mel B Arsodal	Antiparasitic agents
Methenamine hippurate	Hiprex Urex	Other urinary tract agents
Methenamine mandelate	Mandelamine	Other urinary tract agents

(Continues)

Generic	Trade	Family
Methicillin	Celbenin Dimocillin RT Staphcillin	Penicillins
Metronidazole	Flagyl Metric 21 Protostat	Metronidazole
Mezlocillin	Mezlin	Penicillins
Miconazole	Micatin Monistat	Antifungal agents
Minocycline	Minocin Vectrin	Tetracyclines
Moxalactam	Moxam	Cephalosporins
Nafcillin	Nafcil Unipen	Penicillins
Nalidixic acid	Cybis NegGram	Quinolones
Neomycin	Mycifradin	Aminoglycosides
Netilmicin	Netromycin	Aminoglycosides
Niclosamide	Niclocide Yomesan	Antiparasitic agents
Nifurtimox	Bayer 2502 Lampit	Antiparasitic agents
Niridazole	Ambilhar	Antiparasitic agents
Nitrofurantoin	Cyantin Furadantin Macrodantin Trantoin	Other urinary tract agents

Generic	Trade	Family
Norfloxacin	Noroxin	Quinolones
Nystatin	Mycostatin Nilstat	Antifungal agents
Ofloxacin	Floxin	Quinolones
Oxacillin	Bactocill Prostaphlin Resistopen	Penicillins
Oxamniquine	Vansil	Antiparasitic agents
Oxolinic acid	Utibid	Quinolones
Oxytetracycline	Terramycin Uri-Tet	Tetracyclines
Para-aminosalicylic acid	PAS Para Parasal Rezipas	Antimycobacterial agents
Paromomycin	Humatin	Antiparasitic agents
Pefloxacin	Peflacine	Quinolones
Penicillin G	Pentids Pfizerpen	Penicillins
Penicillin G procaine	Crysticillin Duracillin AS Wycillin	Penicillins
Penicillin G sodium + penicillin G procaine	Duracillin FA	Penicillins

(Continues)

Generic	Trade	Family
Penicillin G + phenoxymethyl penicillin	Kesso-pen	Penicillins
Penicillin V potassium (phenoxymethyl penicillin)	Betapen VK Ledercillin VK Penapar VK Pen Vee K Robicillin VK Uticillin VK V-Cillin K Veetids	Penicillins
Pentamidine	Pentam 300 Lomidine	Antiparasitic agents
Phenazopyridine + sulfisoxazole	Azo Gantrisin	Sulfonamide + symptomatic bladder therapy
Phenethicillin	Darcil Maxipen Synicillin	Penicillins
Piperacillin	Pipracil	Penicillins
Piperazine	Antepar	Antiparasitic agents
Polymyxin B	Aerosporin	Polymyxins
Praziquantel	Biltricide	Antiparasitic agents
Primaquine phosphate	Primaquine	Antiparasitic agents
Proguanil	Paludrine	Antiparasitic agents
Pyrantel pamoate	Antiminth	Antiparasitic agents

Generic	Trade	Family
Pyrazinamide	Aldinamid Tebrazid Zinamide	Antimycobacterial agents
Pyrimethamine	Daraprim	Antiparasitic agents
Pyrimethamine sulfadoxine	Fansidar	Antiparasitic agents
Pyrvinium pamoate	Povan	Antiparasitic agents
Quinacrine	Atabrine	Antiparasitic agents
Quinidine gluconate	—	Antiparasitic agents
Quinine sulfate	Quinamm	Antiparasitic agents
Ribavirin	Virazole	Antiviral agents
Rifabutin	Ansamycin	Antimycobacterial agents
Rifampin	Rifadin Rimactane	Antimycobacterial agents
Rifampin-isoniazid	Rifamate	Antimycobacterial agents
Rimantadine	Flumadine	Antiviral agents
Roxithromycin		Macrolides
Silver sulfadiazine	Silvadene	Sulfonamides
Spectinomycin	Trobicin	Aminoglycosides
Spiramycin	—	Macrolides

(Continues)

Generic	Trade	Family
Stibogluconate	Pentostam	Antiparasitic agents
Streptomycin	Strycin Streptolin Streptaquane	Aminoglycosides
Sulfacetamide	Sulamyd	Sulfonamides
Sulfadiazine	Microsulfon	Sulfonamides
Sulfadoxine + pyrimethamine	Fansidar	Antiparasitic agents
Sulfamethizole	Thiosulfil Urobiotic	Sulfonamides
Sulfamethoxazole	Gantanol	Sulfonamides
Sulfanilamide	AVC	Sulfonamides
Sulfaphenazole	—	Sulfonamides
Sulfasalazine	Azulfidine	Sulfonamides
Sulfathiazole/ sulfacetamide/ sulfabenzamide (triple sulfa)	Sultrin Trysul	Sulfonamides
Sulfisoxazole	Gantrisin	Sulfonamides
Sulfisoxazole + phenazopyridine	Azo Gantrisin	Sulfonamides + symptomatic bladder therapy
Suramin	Germanin	Antiparasitic agents
Teicoplanin	Targocid	Vancomycin-like
Temafloxacin	Omniflox	Quinolones

Generic	Trade	Family
Tetracycline	Achromycin Kesso-tetra Panmycin Polycycline Robitet Steclin Sumycin Tetracyn Tetrex	Tetracyclines
Thiabendazole	Mintezol	Antiparasitic agents
Ticarcillin	Ticar	Penicillins
Ticarcillin + clavulanate	Timentin	Penicillins + β- lactamase inhibitors
Tobramycin	Nebcin	Aminoglycosides
Tolnaftate	Tinactin	Antifungal agents
Trifluridine	Viroptic	Antiviral agents
Trimethoprim	Proloprim Trimpex	Trimethoprim
Trimethoprim- sulfamethoxazole	Bactrim Septra	Sulfonamides + trimethoprim
Trisulfapyrimidines	Terfonyl	Sulfonamides
Vancomycin	Vancocin	Vancomycin
Vidarabine	Vira-A	Antiviral agents
Viomycin	Vinactane Viocin	Antimycobacterial agents
Zalcitabine (ddC)	Hivid	Antiretroviral
Zidovudine (AZT)	Retrovir	Antiviral agents

Trade	Generic	Family
Achromycin	Tetracycline	Tetracyclines
Aerosporin	Polymyxin B	Polymyxins
Aldinamid	Pyrazinamide	Antimycobacterial agents
Alferon N	Interferon-α-N3	Antiviral agents
Ampen	Ampicillin	Penicillins
Ambilhar	Niridazole	Antiparasitic agents
Amcill	Ampicillin	Penicillins
Amikin	Amikacin	Aminoglycosides
Amoxil	Amoxicillin	Penicillins
Ancef	Cefazolin	Cephalosporins
Ancobon	Flucytosine	Antifungal agents
Anspor	Cephradine	Cephalosporins
Antiminth	Pyrantel pamoate	Antiparasitic agents
Apace	Cefotetan	Cephalosporins
Aralen	Chloroquine	Antiparasitic agents
Arsobal	Melarsoprol B	Antiparasitic agents
Atabrine	Quinacrine	Antiparasitic agents
A/T/S	Erythromycin	Erythromycins
Augmentin	Amoxicillin + clavulanate	β-Lactamase inhibitors + penicillins
Aureomycin	Chlortetracycline	Tetracyclines

Trade	Generic	Family
AVC	Sulfanilamide	Sulfonamides
Avlosulfon	Dapsone	Antimycobacterial agents
Azactam	Aztreonam	Other β-Lactams
Azlin	Azlocillin	Penicillins
Azo Gantrisin	Sulfisoxazole + phenazopyridine	Sulfonamides + symptomatic bladder therapy
Azulfidine	Sulfasalazine	Sulfonamides
Bactocill	Oxacillin	Penicillins
Bactrim	Trimethoprim-sulfamethoxazole	Sulfonamides + trimethoprim
Bayer 2502	Nifurtimox	Antiparasitic agents
Benzamycin	Erythromycin	Erythromycins
Betapen VK	Penicillin V potassium	Penicillins
Biaxin	Clarithromycin	Macrolides
Bicillin	Benzathine penicillin G	Penicillins
Biltricide	Praziquantel	Antiparasitic agents
Bitin	Bithionol	Antiparasitic agents
Canesten	Clotrimazole	Antifungal agents
Capastat	Capreomycin	Antimycobacterial agents
Ceclor	Cefaclor	Cephalosporins

(Continues)

Trade	Generic	Family
Cefadyl	Cephapirin	Cephalosporins
Cefatrexail	Cephapirin	Cephalosporins
Cefizox	Ceftizoxime	Cephalosporins
Cefmax	Cefmenoxime	Cephalosporins
Cefobid	Cefoperazone	Cephalosporins
Cefomonil	Cefsulodin	Cephalosporins
Cefotan	Cefotetan	Cephalosporins
Ceftin	Cefuroxime axetil	Cephalosporins
Celbenin	Methicillin	Penicillins
Chloromycetin	Chloramphenicol	Chloramphenicol
Cipro	Ciprofloxacin	Quinolones
Claforan	Cefotaxime	Cephalosporins
Cleocin	Clindamycin	Lincosamides
Coactin	Amdinocillin	Penicillins
Colymycin M	Colistimethate	Polymyxins
Colymycin S	Colistin	Polymyxins
Cosmosin	Cefuzonam	Cephalosporins
Crysticillin	Penicillin G procaine	Penicillins
Cyantin	Nitrofurantoin	Other urinary tract agents
Cybis	Nalidixic acid	Quinolones
Cyclapen	Cyclacillin	Penicillins

Trade	Generic	Family
Cytovene	Ganciclovir	Antivirals
Daraprim	Pyrimethamine	Antiparasitic agents
Darcil	Phenethicillin	Penicillins
Declomycin	Demeclocycline	Tetracyclines
Dendrid	Idoxuridine	Antiviral agents
Diflucan	Fluconazole	Antifungal agents
Dimocillin RT	Methicillin	Penicillins
Doxy II	Doxycycline	Tetracyclines
Doxychel	Doxycycline	Tetracyclines
Doyle	Aspoxicillin	Penicillins
Duracillin AS	Penicillin G procaine	Penicillins
Duracillin FA	Penicillin G sodium + penicillin G procaine	Penicillins
Duricef	Cefadroxil	Cephalosporins
Dycill	Dicloxacillin	Penicillins
Dynapen	Dicloxacillin	Penicillins
E-mycin	Erythromycin	Erythromycins
E.E.S.	Erythromycin ethylsuccinate	Erythromycins
ERYC	Erythromycin	Erythromycins
Erycette	Erythromycin	Erythromycins

(Continues)

Trade	Generic	Family
Eryderm	Erythromycin	Erythromycins
Erygel	Erythromycin	Erythromycins
Erymax	Erythromycin	Erythromycins
Ery-Ped	Erythromycin ethylsuccinate	Erythromycins
Ery-Tab	Erythromycin	Erythromycins
Erythrocin	Erythromycin stearate	Erythromycins
Erythrocin lactobionate	Erythromycin lactobionate	Erythromycins
ESP	Erythromycin ethylsuccinate + sulfisoxazole	Erythromycins + sulfonamides
Ethril	Erythromycin	Erythromycins
ETS - 2%	Erythromycin	Erythromycins
Fansidar	Pyrimethamine + sulfadoxine	Antiparasitic agents
Flagyl	Metronidazole	Metronidazole
Floxapen	Flucloxacillin	Penicillins
Floxin	Ofloxacin	Quinolones
Flumadine	Rimantadine	Antiviral agents
Flumarin	Flumoxef	Cephalosporins
Fortaz	Ceftazidime	Cephalosporins
Foscavir	Foscarnet	Antiviral agents

Trade	Generic	Family
Fosmicin	Fosfomycin	
Fulvicin P-G	Griseofulvin	Antifungal agents
Fulvicin U-F	Griseofulvin	Antifungal agents
Fungizone	Amphotericin B	Antifungal agents
Furadantin	Nitrofurantoin	Other urinary tract agents
Furamide	Diloxanide furoate	Antiparasitic agents
Gantanol	Sulfamethoxazole	Sulfonamides
Gantrisin	Sulfisoxazole	Sulfonamides
Garamycin	Gentamicin	Aminoglycosides
Geocillin	Carbenicillin indanyl sodium	Penicillins
Geopen	Carbenicillin	Penicillins
Germanin	Suramin	Antiparasitic agents
Grifulvin V	Griseofulvin	Antifungal agents
Gris-PEG	Griseofulvin	Antifungal agents
Grisactin	Griseofulvin	Antifungal agents
Herplex	Idoxuridine	Antiviral agents
Hetrazan	Diethylcarbamazine	Antiparasitic agents
Hiprex	Methenamine hippurate	Other urinary tract agents
Humatin	Paromomycin	Antiparasitic agents

(Continues)

Trade	Generic	Family
Hyzyd	Isoniazid	Antimycobacterial agents
Ilosone	Erythromycin estolate	Erythromycins
Ilotycin	Erythromycin	Erythromycins
Ilotycin gluceptate	Erythromycin gluceptate	Erythromycins
INH	Isoniazid	Antimycobacterial agents
Intron A	Interferon-α-2B, recombinant	Antiviral agents
Kafocin	Cephaloglycin	Cephalosporins
Kantrex	Kanamycin	Aminoglycosides
Keflex	Cephalexin	Cephalosporins
Keflin	Cephalothin	Cephalosporins
Kefurox	Cefuroxime	Cephalosporins
Kefzol	Cefazolin	Cephalosporins
Keiperazon	Cefbuperazone	Cephalosporins
Kesso-mycin	Erythromycin	Erythromycins
Kesso-pen	Penicillin G + phenoxymethyl penicillin	Penicillins
Kesso-tetra	Tetracycline	Tetracyclines
Lampit	Nifurtimox	Antiparasitic agents

Trade	Generic	Family
Lamprene	Clofazimine	Antimycobacterial agents
Lariam	Mefloquine	Antiparasitic agents
Larotid	Amoxicillin	Penicillins
Ledercillin VK	Penicillin V potassium	Penicillins
Lomidine	Pentamidine	Antiparasitic agents
Lorothidol	Bithionol	Antiparasitic agents
Lotrimin	Clotrimazole	Antifungal agents
Macrodantin	Nitrofurantoin	Other urinary tract agents
Mandelamine	Methenamine mandelate	Other urinary tract agents
Mandol	Cefamandole	Cephalosporins
Maxipen	Phenethicillin	Penicillins
Mectizan	Ivermectin	Antiparasitic agents
Mefoxin	Cefoxitin	Cephalosporins
Meicelin	Cefminox	Cephalosporins
Mel B	Melarsoprol B	Antiparasitic agents
Metric 21	Metronidazole	Metronidazole
Mezlin	Mezlocillin	Penicillins
Micatin	Miconazole	Antifungal agents
Microsulfon	Sulfadiazine	Sulfonamides

(Continues)

Trade	Generic	Family
Minocin	Minocycline	Tetracyclines
Mintezol	Thiabendazole	Antiparasitic agents
Monocid	Cefonicid	Cephalosporins
Monistat	Miconazole	Antifungal agents
Moxam	Moxalactam	Cephalosporins
Myambutol	Ethambutol	Antimycobacterial agents
Mycelex	Clotrimazole	Antifungal agents
Mycifradin	Neomycin	Aminoglycosides
Mycostatin	Nystatin	Antifungal agents
Microsulfon	Sulfadiazine	Sulfonamides
Nafcil	Nafcillin	Penicillins
Nebcin	Tobramycin	Aminoglycosides
NegGram	Nalidixic acid	Quinolones
Netromycin	Netilmicin	Aminoglycosides
Niadox	Isoniazid	Antimycobacterial agents
Niclocide	Niclosamide	Antiparasitic agents
Niconyl	Isoniazid	Antimycobacterial agents
Nilstat	Nystatin	Antifungal agents
Nizoral	Ketoconazole	Antifungal agents

Trade	Generic	Family
Noroxin	Norfloxacin	Quinolones
Nydrazid	Isoniazid	Antimycobacterial agents
Omniflox	Temafloxacin	Quinolones
Omnipen	Ampicillin	Penicillins
Omnipen-N	Ampicillin	Penicillins
Oxamycin	Cycloserine	Antimycobacterial agents
PAS	Para-aminosalicylic acid	Antimycobacterial agents
Paludrine	Proguanil	Antiparasitic agent
Panimycin	Dibekacin	Aminoglycosides
Panmycin	Tetracycline	Tetracyclines
Pansporin	Cefotiam	Cephalosporins
Panthrone	Amithiozone (thiacetazone)	Antimycobacterial agents
Para	Para-aminosalicylic acid	Antimycobacterial agents
Parasal	Para-aminosalicylic acid	Antimycobacterial agents
Pathocil	Dicloxacillin	Penicillins
Pediazole	Erythromycin ethylsuccinate + sulfisoxazole	Erythromycins + sulfonamides

(Continues)

Trade	Generic	Family
Peflacine	Pefloxacin	Quinolones
Pen Vee K	Penicillin V potassium	Penicillins
PenA	Ampicillin	Penicillins
Penapar VK	Penicillin V potassium	Penicillins
Penbritin	Ampicillin	Penicillins
Pensyn	Ampicillin	Penicillins
Pentam 300	Pentamidine	Antiparasitic agents
Pentids	Penicillin G	Penicillins
Pentostam	Stibogluconate	Antiparasitic agents
Permapen	Benzathine penicillin G	Penicillins
Pfizerpen	Penicillin G	Penicillins
Pipracil	Piperacillin	Penicillins
Polycillin	Ampicillin	Penicillins
Polycillin-N	Ampicillin	Penicillins
Polycillin-PRB	Ampicillin probenecid	Penicillins
Polycycline	Tetracycline	Tetracyclines
Polymox	Amoxicillin	Penicillins
Povan	Pyrvinium pamoate	Antiparasitic agents
Precef	Ceforanide	Cephalosporins
Primaquine	Primaquine phosphate	Antiparasitic agents
Primaxin	Imipenem + cilastatin	Carbapenems

Trade	Generic	Family
Principen	Ampicillin	Penicillins
Probampacin	Ampicillin	Penicillins
Proloprim	Trimethoprim	Trimethoprim
Prostaphlin	Oxacillin	Penicillins
Protostat	Metronidazole	Metronidazole
Pyopen	Carbenicillin	Penicillins
Quinamm	Quinine sulfate	Antiparasitic agents
Resistopen	Oxacillin	Penicillins
Retrovir	Zidovudine (AZT)	Antiviral agents
Rezipas	Para-aminosalicylic acid	Antimycobacterial agents
Rifadin	Rifampin	Antimycobacterial agents
Rifamate	Rifampin-isoniazid	Antimycobacterial agents
Rifabutin	Ansamycin	Antimycobacterial agents
Rimactane	Rifampin	Antimycobacterial agents
Robamox	Amoxicillin	Penicillins
Robicillin VK	Penicillin V potassium	Penicillins
Robimycin	Erythromycin	Erythromycins

(Continues)

Trade	Generic	Family
Robitet	Tetracycline	Tetracyclines
Rocephin	Ceftriaxone	Cephalosporins
Roferon-A	Interferon-α-2A, recombinant	Antiviral agents
Septra	Trimethoprim-sulfamethoxazole	Sulfonamides and trimethoprim
Seromycin	Cycloserine	Antimycobacterial agents
Silvadene	Silver sulfadiazine	Sulfonamides
Spectrobid	Bacampicillin	Penicillins
Sporanox	Itraconazole	Antifungal agents
Staphcillin	Methicillin	Penicillins
Steclin	Tetracycline	Tetracyclines
Stoxil	Idoxuridine	Antiviral agents
Streptaquane	Streptomycin	Aminoglycosides
Streptolin	Streptomycin	Aminoglycosides
Strycin	Streptomycin	Aminoglycosides
Sulamyd	Sulfacetamide	Sulfonamides
Sulfamylon	Mafenide	Sulfonamides
Sulperazone	Cefoperazone + sulbactam	Cephalosporines + β-Lactamase inhibitors

Trade	Generic	Family
Sultrin	Sulfathiazole/ sulfacetamide/ sulfabenzamide (triple sulfa)	Sulfonamides
Sumycin	Tetracycline	Tetracyclines
Suncefal	Cefpiramide	Cephalosporins
Supen	Ampicillin	Penicillins
Suprax	Cefixime	Cephalosporins
Symmetrel	Amantadine	Antiviral agents
Synicillin	Phenethicillin	Penicillins
Targocid	Teicoplanin	Vancomycin-like
Tazicef	Ceftazidime	Cephalosporins
Tazidime	Ceftazidime	Cephalosporins
Tegopen	Cloxacillin	Penicillins
Terfonyl	Trisulfapyrimidines	Sulfonamides
Terramycin	Oxytetracycline	Tetracyclines
Tetracyn	Tetracycline	Tetracyclines
Tetrex	Tetracycline	Tetracyclines
Thiosulfil	Sulfamethizole	Sulfonamides
Tibione	Amithiozone (thiacetazone)	Antimycobacterial agents

(Continues)

Trade	Generic	Family
Ticar	Ticarcillin	Penicillins
Timentin	Ticarcillin + clavulanate	Penicillins + β-lactamase inhibitors
Tinactin	Tolnaftate	Antifungal agents
Totacillin	Ampicillin	Penicillins
Trantoin	Nitrofurantoin	Other urinary tract agents
Trecator-SC	Ethionamide	Antimycobacterial agents
Trimox	Amoxicillin	Penicillins
Trimpex	Trimethoprim	Trimethoprim
Trobicin	Spectinomycin	Aminoglycosides
Trojacillin-Plus	Ampicillin probenecid	Penicillins
Trysul	Sulfathiazole/ sulfacetamide/ sulfabenzamide (triple sulfa)	Sulfonamides
Unasyn	Ampicillin + sulbactam	β-Lactamase inhibitors + penicillins
Unipen	Nafcillin	Penicillins
Urex	Methenamine hippurate	Other urinary tract agents
Uri-tet	Oxytetracycline	Tetracyclines

Trade	Generic	Family
Urobiotic	Sulfamethizole	Sulfonamides
Utibid	Oxolinic acid	Quinolones
Uticillin VK	Penicillin V potassium	Penicillins
V-Cillin K	Penicillin V potassium	Penicillins
Vancocin	Vancomycin	Vancomycin
Vansil	Oxamniquine	Antiparasitic agents
Vectrin	Minocycline	Tetracycline
Veetids	Penicillin V potassium	Penicillins
Velosef	Cephradine	Cephalosporins
Veracillin	Dicloxacillin	Penicillins
Vermox	Mebendazole	Antiparasitic agents
Versapen	Hetacillin	Penicillins
Versapen K	Hetacillin	Penicillins
Vibramycin	Doxycycline	Tetracyclines
Videx	Didanosine (dideoxyinosine [ddl])	Antiviral agents
Vinactane	Viomycin	Antimycobacterial agents
Viocin	Viomycin	Antimycobacterial agents
Vira-A	Vidarabine	Antiviral agents

(Continues)

Trade	Generic	Family
Virazole	Ribavirin	Antiviral agents
Viroptic	Trifluridine	Antiviral agents
Wyamycin S	Erythromycin stearate	Erythromycins
Wycillin	Penicillin G procaine	Penicillins
Yodoxin	Iodoquinol	Antiparasitic agents
Yomesan	Niclosamide	Antiparasitic agents
Zefazone	Cefmetazole	Cephalosporins
Zentel	Albendazole	Antiparasitic agents
Zinacef	Cefuroxime	Cephalosporins
Zinamide	Pyrazinamide	Antimycobacterial agents
Zithromax	Azithromycin	Macrolide
Zovirax	Acyclovir	Antiviral agents

Index